INFUSED
Water

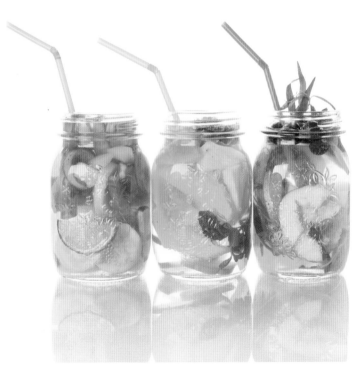

INFUSED
Water

75 Simple and Delicious Recipes to Keep
You and Your Family Healthy and Happy

DALILA TARHUNI

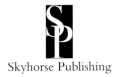

Skyhorse Publishing

Skyhorse Publishing books may be purchased in bulk at special discounts
for sales promotion, corporate gifts, fund-raising, or educational purposes.
Special editions can also be created to specifications. For details, contact the
Special Sales Department, Skyhorse Publishing, 307 West 36th Street, 11th
Floor, New York, NY 10018 or info@skyhorsepublishing.com.

Skyhorse® and Skyhorse Publishing® are registered trademarks of
Skyhorse Publishing, Inc.®, a Delaware corporation.

Visit our website at www.skyhorsepublishing.com.

10 9 8 7 6 5 4 3 2 1

Library of Congress Cataloging-in-Publication Data is available on file.

Cover design by Jane Sheppard
Cover photograph by Dalila Tarhuni

Print ISBN: 978-1-5107-0898-3
Ebook ISBN: 978-1-5107-0900-3

Printed in China

Contents

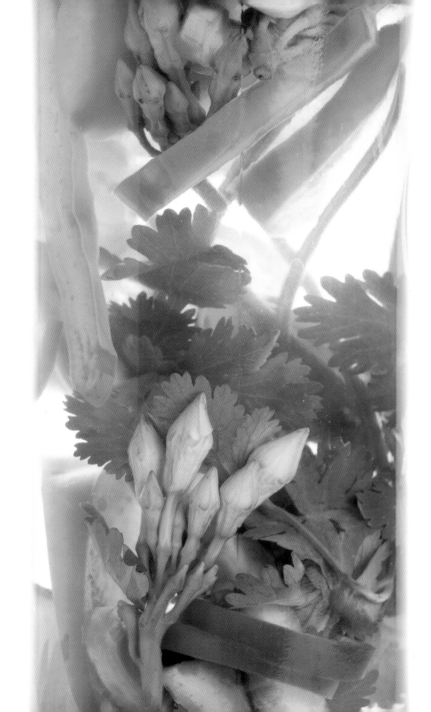

Why Infuse Water

We all know our bodies need water to function. Hydration is essential for good health and glowing skin, yet most of us are not getting enough. While the recommended quantity of eight glasses of water per day is debatable as it depends on various factors such as body size, weather, and exercise levels, it is absolutely important that we stay hydrated. Without a doubt one of the trendiest (and tastiest) ways to do this is infused water. Although it has been around for a very long time, in recent years its popularity has soared among health enthusiasts—and for good reason! Infused water is delicious, full of beneficial nutrients, easy to make, and a healthier substitute for sugary beverages. If you find regular water somewhat boring, simply adding a slice of lemon or a sprig of fresh mint will give it a more pleasant and refreshing taste. Or you can get creative and experiment with combining your favorite fruits and veggies to derive a plethora of flavors.

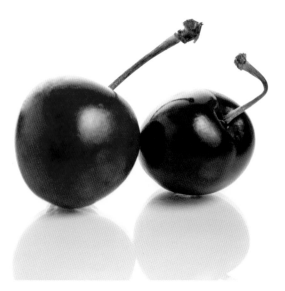

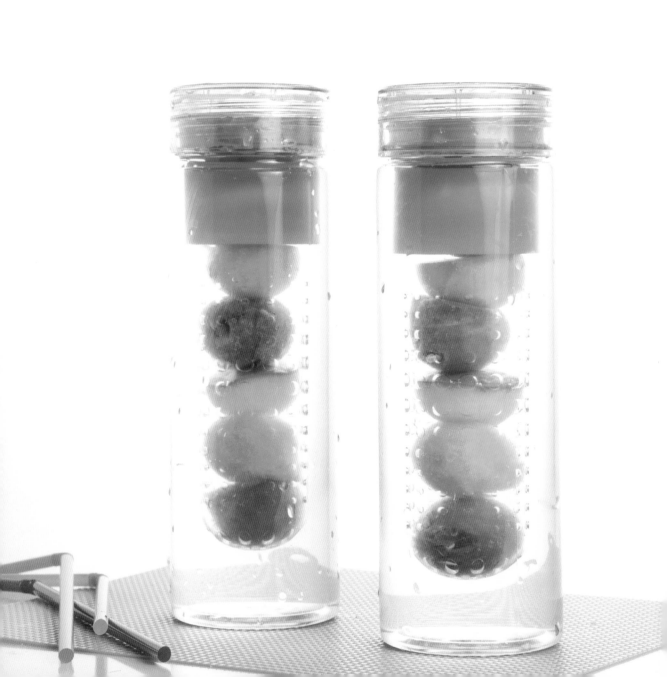

Tips for Infusing

- Whenever possible, choose organic produce; wash well under cold, running water to remove chemicals, pesticides, and other residues.
- For a more robust flavor, crush fresh herbs with a muddler or a wooden spoon before adding to the water.
- Water infused with an unpeeled citrus fruit will start tasting bitter after a few hours, so it is best to peel it if you don't plan to drink the water right away.
- Use cold or room temperature filtered or spring water. If you prefer sparkling water, infuse the ingredients in half of the recommended quantity water, then add the remaining just before serving.
- Ideally, infuse the water in glass vessels, such as jars and pitchers. The special infuser water bottles and pitchers are useful, but not a must-have. A tea infuser is useful for loose herbs and spices.
- Always refrigerate the infused water within one to two hours of making it to prevent bacterial growth.

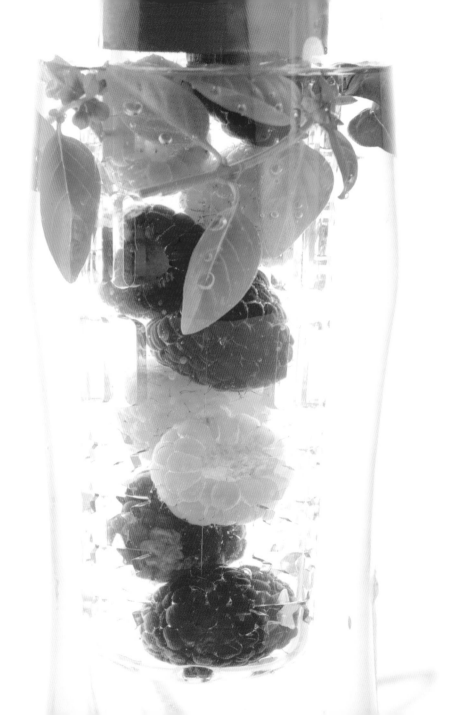

How to Infuse Water

Quick Infusion

- Select the fruits, vegetables, and herbs you would like to infuse your water with. Citrus fruit, watermelon, strawberries, cucumbers, mint, and basil, are most suitable for quick infusion as they will flavor the water almost right away.
- Thinly slice, dice, or spiralize the fruits and/or vegetables and place in a glass or water bottle.
- If you are using fresh herbs, mash them with the help of a muddler or a wooden spoon prior to stirring in.
- If you wish, you may add a little sweetener of choice.
- Fill the glass with water, stir, and enjoy right away.

Slow Infusion

- Select the fruits, vegetables, herbs, and spices you would like to infuse your water with.
- Slice, dice, or spiralize the fruits and veggies and place in an infuser water bottle, lidded jar, or a pitcher; add herbs and spices, and sweetener if using.
- Fill with water, cover, and refrigerate for 2 to 4 hours or overnight before serving.
- You may refill a few times with fresh water if you wish.
- The infused water will keep in the refrigerator for 2 to 3 days, but it may be a good idea to strain and discard the fruit and veggies if they start looking soggy. Strawberries and watermelons are best discarded after a few hours of soaking.

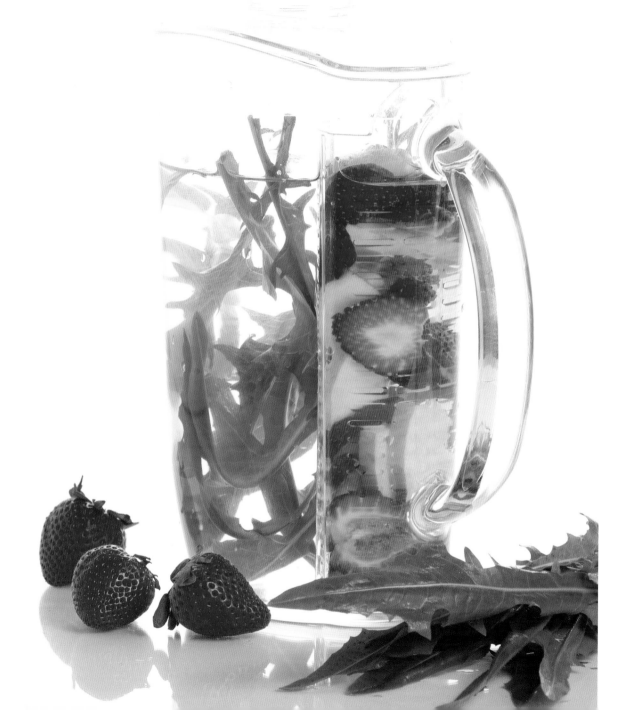

Apple, Dandelion, and Strawberry

Servings: 6–8
Prep Time: 5 minutes
Infusing Time: 3–4 hours

Ingredients:

1 Granny Smith apple, cored and sliced
⅔ cup strawberries, hulled and sliced
A few lemon or lime slices
½ bunch (1 handful) fresh dandelion greens*
6–8 cups filtered or spring water
Ice cubes, to serve

Directions:

Add the apple, strawberry, lemon or lime slices, and dandelion leaves to the pitcher. Fill with water and place in the fridge for about 3–4 hours to let the flavors infuse.

Serve with ice and use within 1–2 days.

TIP
*If fresh dandelion greens are not available, substitute with arugula or watercress, or infuse cold brewed dandelion leaves and root tea with the fruit.

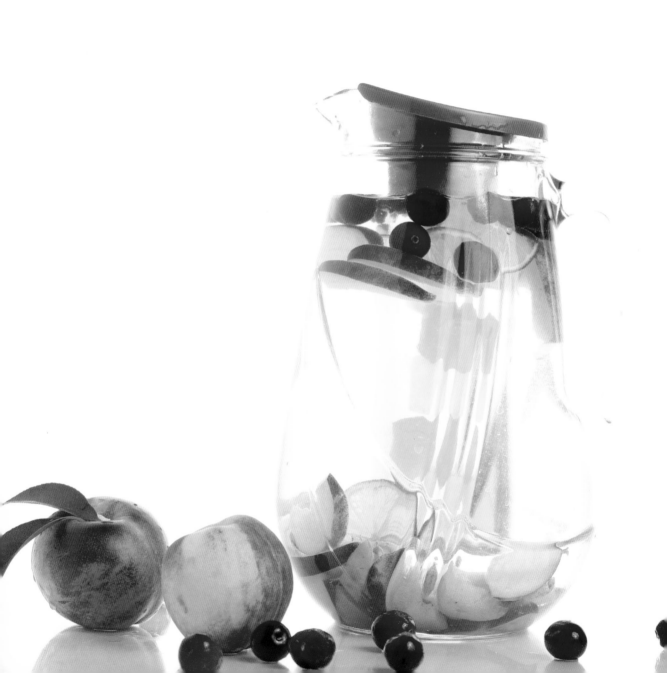

Apricot, Nectarine, Peach, and Cranberries

SERVINGS: 6–8
PREP TIME: 10 MINUTES
INFUSING TIME: 3–4 HOURS

Ingredients:

1 nectarine, pitted and sliced
1 white peach, pitted and sliced
2 apricots, pitted and sliced
⅓ cup fresh or frozen cranberries
2–3 lime or lemon slices
6–8 cups filtered or spring water
Ice cubes, to serve

Directions:

Add sliced fruit to a pitcher and fill with water.

Refrigerate for 3–4 hours or overnight. Serve with ice. You may refill with water 2–3 times. Best used within 2–3 days.

TIP
Add a vanilla pod to the water before infusing.

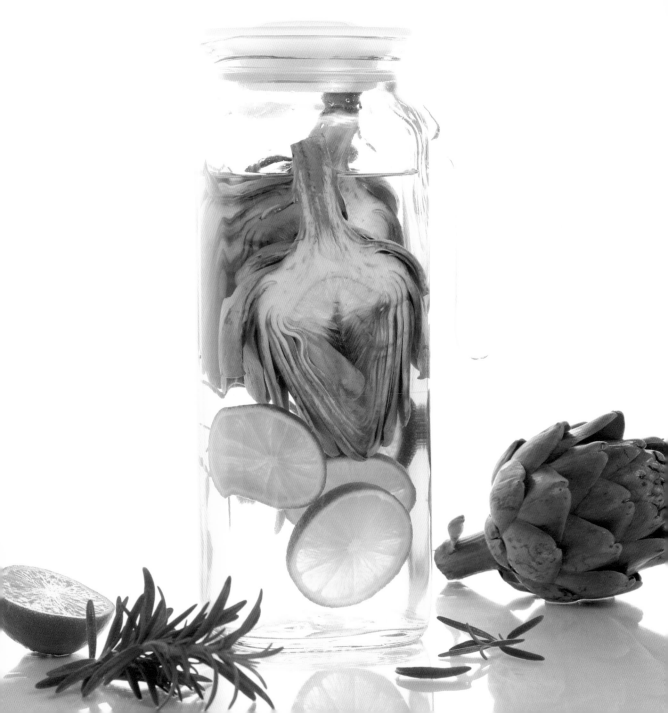

Artichoke, Lime, and Rosemary

SERVINGS: **4–6**
PREP TIME: **10** MINUTES
INFUSING TIME: **3–4** HOURS

Ingredients:

1 small artichoke, trimmed and
   cut in half lengthwise
1 sprig rosemary
1 lime, thinly sliced
2–3 (2-inch) pieces peeled raw
   sugar cane, to taste★
4–6 cups filtered or spring water

Directions:

In a large jar or another glass container, combine artichoke, rosemary, lime, and sugar cane; fill with water and refrigerate overnight.

TIP
★Substitute raw sugar cane with another sweetener of choice.

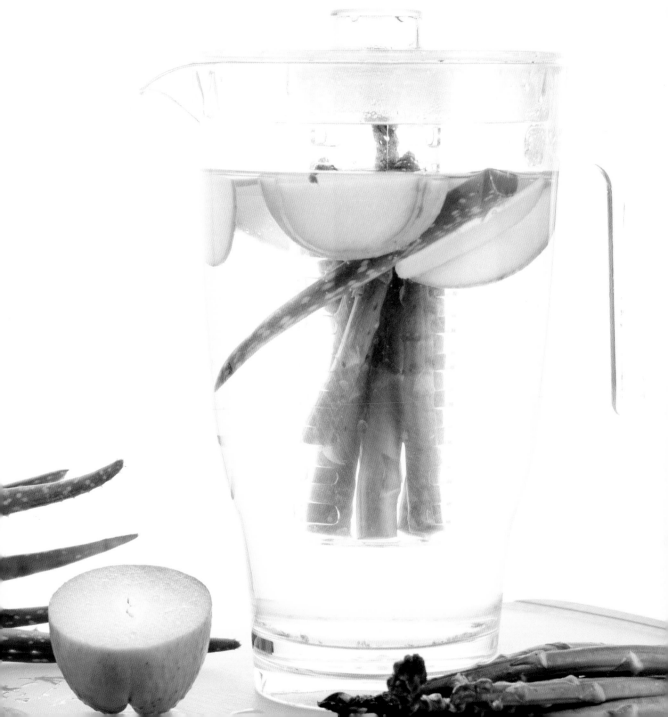

Asparagus, Chayote, and Aloe Vera

SERVINGS: **6–8**
PREP TIME: **10** MINUTES
INFUSING TIME: **3–4** HOURS, PREFERABLY OVERNIGHT

Ingredients:

1 fresh aloe vera leaf★
2 tablespoons freshly squeezed
   lemon juice
½ cup filtered or spring water
1 chayote, thinly sliced
4 stalks asparagus, cut into
   2-inch pieces
Sweetener of choice, to taste
   (optional)
6–8 cups filtered or spring water

Directions:

Using a sharp knife, cut the aloe vera leaf close to the base and place in a jar; let stand for about 10 minutes to allow the sap to ooze out. Wash the leaf, place it on a cutting board flat side up, and slice off the top lengthwise. Scrape out the translucent gel with a spoon; measure 2 tablespoons gel, rinse, add to a blender, together with the lemon juice and ½ cup water; pulse until well-blended together, then pour into a pitcher or a large jar. Add chayote and asparagus, and fill the pitcher with water. Refrigerate for 2–4 hours before serving.

TIP
★Do not immerse a whole aloe vera leaf in your water as shown in the photo—this was only used for styling purposes. Use fresh aloe vera gel as directed in the recipe, or substitute water with shop-bought aloe vera water.

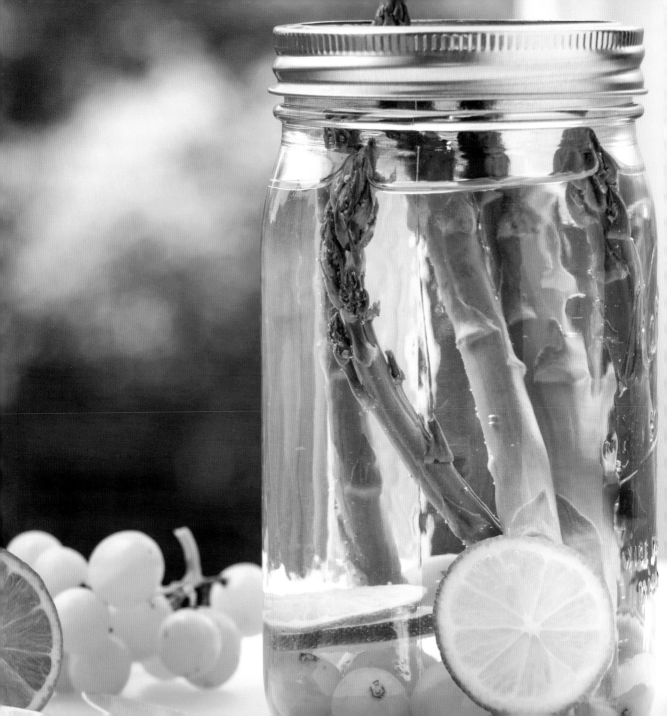

Asparagus, Green Grapes, and Lime

SERVINGS: **4–6**
PREP TIME: **5–7** MINUTES
INFUSING TIME: OVERNIGHT

Ingredients:

4–5 spears young asparagus,
   cut in half
½ cup seedless green grapes,
   cut in half
½ lime, thinly sliced
1 sprig fresh marjoram★
4–6 cups filtered or spring water
Ice cubes, to serve

Directions:

In a large jar, combine all of the ingredients; fill the jar with water and let infuse overnight.

You may refill with water a few times. Use within 3 days.

TIP
★Substitute fresh marjoram with thyme or savory.

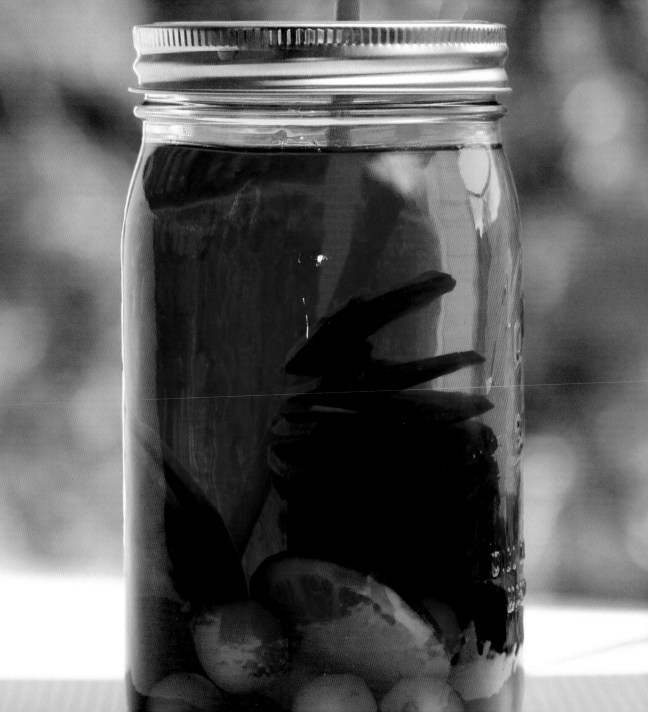

Beets, Green Grapes, and Red Grapes

SERVINGS: 6–8
PREP TIME: 10 MINUTES
INFUSING TIME: 3–4 HOURS

Ingredients:

½ cup seedless green grapes,
   cut in half
½ cup seedless red grapes,
   cut in half
1 small red beet, peeled and
   thinly sliced
½ lime, sliced
6–8 cups filtered or spring water
Ice cubes, to serve

Directions:

Place all of the ingredients in a pitcher or a large jar; fill with water and chill for about 3–4 hours. Use within 3 days.

TIP
For a refreshing twist, add a couple of sprigs of fresh basil.

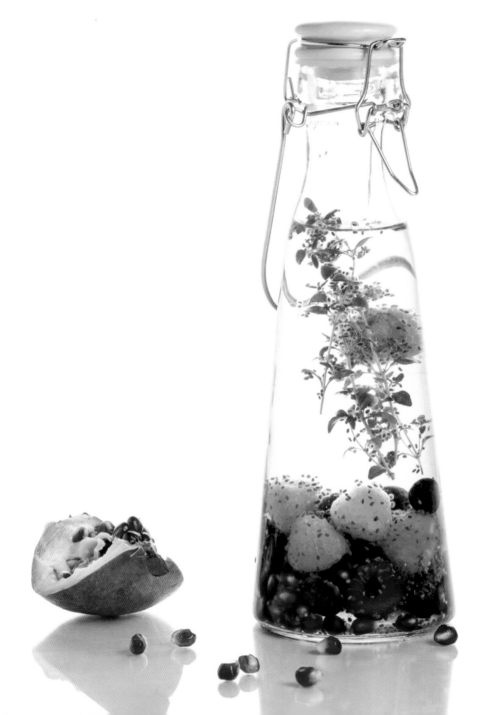

Berries, Pomegranate, Thyme, and Chia Seeds

SERVINGS: **4–6**
PREP TIME: **5** MINUTES
INFUSING TIME: **2–3** HOURS

Ingredients:

2 teaspoons chia seeds
4–6 cups filtered or spring water
1 cup fresh or frozen mixed berries
⅓ cup pomegranate seeds
1 tablespoon fresh lemon juice
3–4 sprigs fresh thyme
Sweetener of choice, to taste

Directions:

Add chia seeds to a large jar or another glass container, add 1 cup of water, and stir to combine. Add berries, pomegranate seeds, lemon juice, thyme, and sweetener; fill the jar with water and refrigerate for 2–3 hours until the flavors have infused.

Use within 2 days.

TIP
Chia seeds will swell up and form clumps, so stir or shake well before serving.

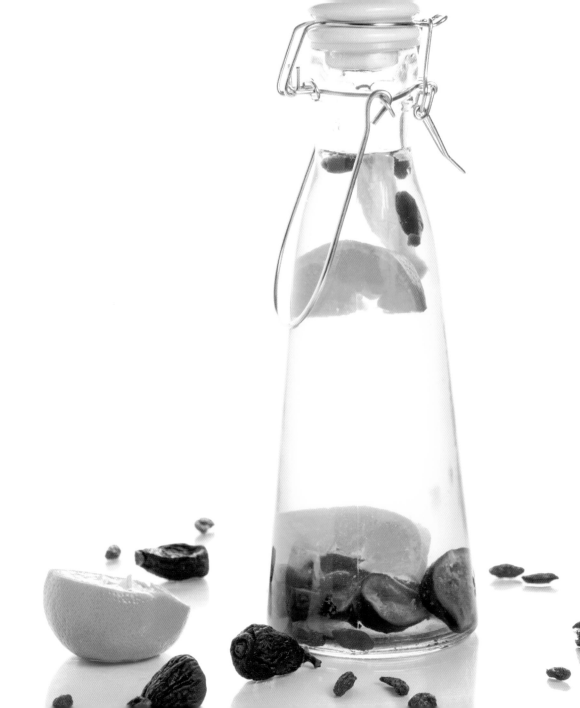

Black Mission Figs, Mandarin Orange, and Cranberries

SERVINGS: 6–8
PREP TIME: 5 MINUTES
INFUSING TIME: OVERNIGHT

Ingredients:

4–5 dried black mission figs,
  cut in half lengthwise
1–2 tablespoons dried goji berries*
2 tablespoons dried cranberries
1 (1½-inch) piece cinnamon bark
  (optional)
1 mandarin orange, sliced
6–8 cups filtered or spring water
A squeeze of lemon juice, to serve

Directions:

Add all ingredients to a pitcher or a large glass jar; fill with water and refrigerate overnight. Serve with a squeeze of lemon juice.

Use within 3 days.

TIP
*If dried goji berries are not available, substitute with dried cranberries or currants.

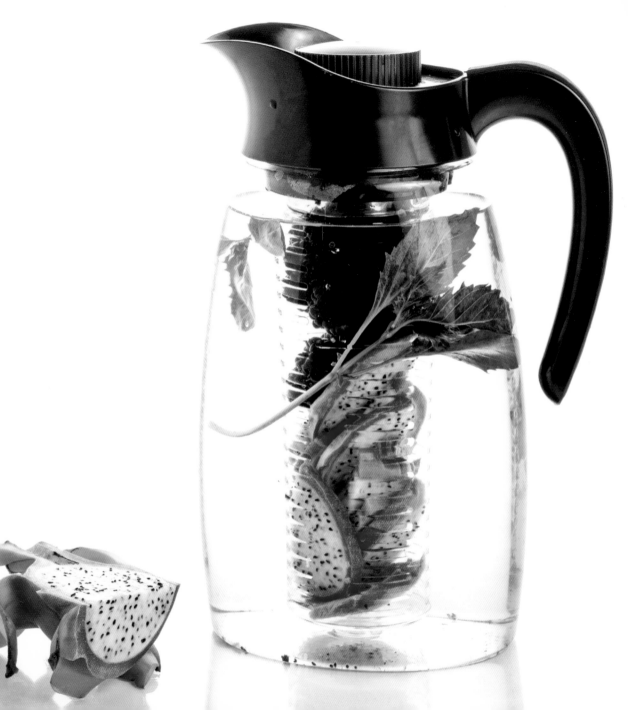

Blackberries, Dragon Fruit, and Purple Basil

SERVINGS: 6–8
PREP TIME: 5 MINUTES
INFUSING TIME: 3–4 HOURS

Ingredients:

½ dragon fruit,* trimmed and sliced
½ cup blackberries
2–3 sprigs purple basil
1 tablespoon chia seeds (optional)
6–8 cups filtered or spring water
Ice cubes, to serve

Directions:

In a pitcher, combine dragon fruit, blackberries, purple basil, and chia seeds, if using.

Fill the pitcher with water and refrigerate for 3–4 hours. Stir before serving.

Use within 2 days.

TIP
*If dragon fruit is not available, substitute with peeled and sliced kiwi.

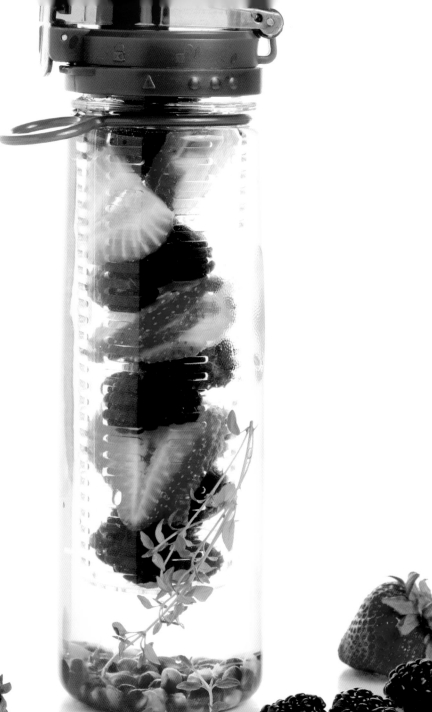
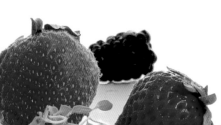

Blackberry, Strawberry, and Pomegranate

SERVINGS: 4–6
PREP TIME: 10 MINUTES
INFUSING TIME: 3–4 HOURS

Ingredients:

¼ cup blackberries
2–3 strawberries, hulled and sliced
2–3 tablespoons pomegranate seeds
A few sprigs fresh thyme★
6–8 cups filtered or spring water

Directions:

Combine all of the ingredients in an infuser water bottle or a mason jar and fill with water. Chill for 2–3 hours before serving.

Use within 2 days.

TIP
★Substitute thyme with fresh oregano or marjoram.

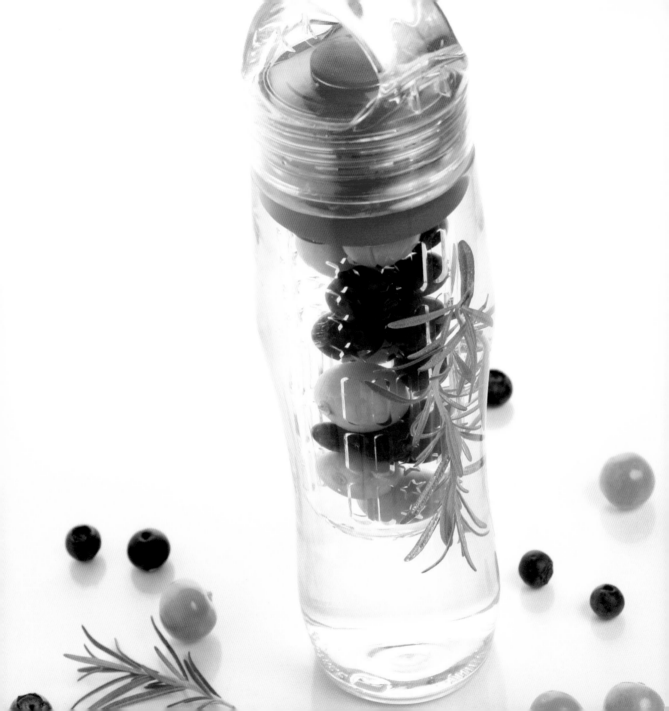

Blueberries, Golden Berries, and Rosemary

SERVINGS: **2–3**
PREP TIME: **5** MINUTES
INFUSING TIME: OVERNIGHT

Ingredients:

¼ cup blueberries
¼ cup golden berries (cape
   gooseberries),* cut in half
1 small sprig rosemary
Sweetener of choice, to taste
2–3 cups filtered or spring water

Directions:

Combine blueberries, golden berries, and rosemary in an infuser water bottle or mason jar. Add sweetener to taste and fill with water; seal tightly and refrigerate overnight. You may refill with water and let infuse for a few hours. Use within 2 days.

TIP
*Substitute golden berries with sliced tomatillos or gooseberries (or use only blueberries).

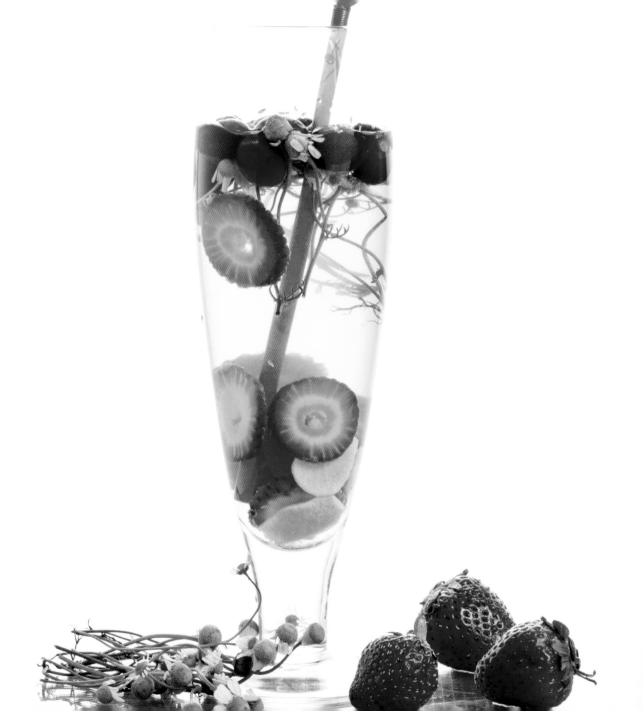

Chamomile, Cranberry, Strawberry, and Ginger

SERVINGS: 4–6
PREP TIME: 5 MINUTES
INFUSING TIME: 1–3 HOURS

Ingredients:

¼ cup fresh or frozen cranberries
½ cup strawberries, hulled and sliced
1 (1-inch) piece ginger, peeled and sliced
Sweetener of choice, to taste
1 tablespoon fresh chamomile flowers (or 1 teaspoon dried)★
4–6 cups filtered or spring water

Directions:

In a large jar, combine cranberries, strawberries, ginger, and sweetener, if using; place chamomile flowers in a tea ball infuser and add to the jar. Fill the jar with water and chill for 2–4 hours.

Use within 2 days.

TIP
★Substitute chamomile flowers with 1 bag chamomile tea.

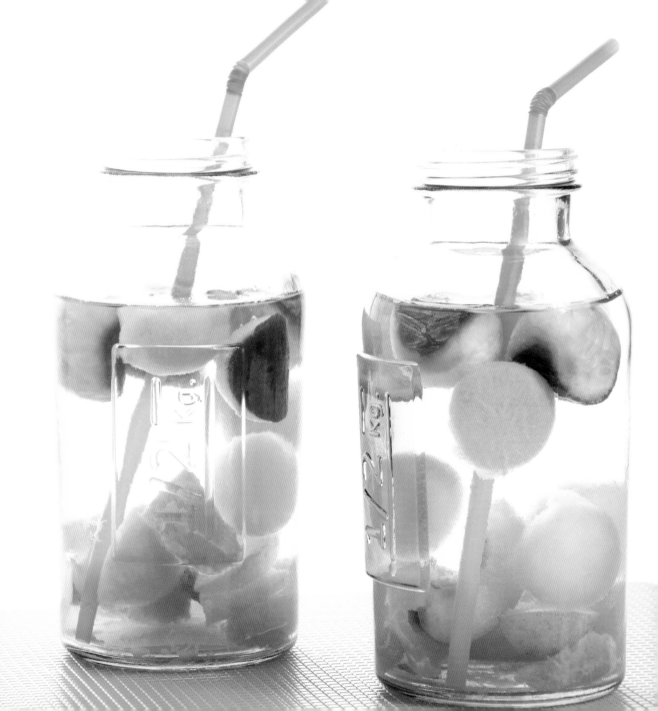

Cantaloupe, Honeydew, Cucumber, Apricot, and Mandarin Orange

SERVINGS: 6–8
PREP TIME: 10 MINUTES
INFUSING TIME: 3–4 HOURS

Ingredients:

½ cup cantaloupe, sliced
½ cup honeydew, sliced
½ cup cucumber, sliced
2 apricots, pitted and sliced
1 mandarin orange, segmented
6–8 cups filtered or spring water★
Ice cubes, to serve

Directions:

Place all ingredients in a pitcher and fill with water.

Chill for 2–4 hours. You may refill with water 2–4 times. Keep refrigerated for up to 2 days.

TIP
★To make the infusion with sparkling water, infuse the fruit in 4–5 cups sparkling water for 2–4 hours and add the remaining just before serving.

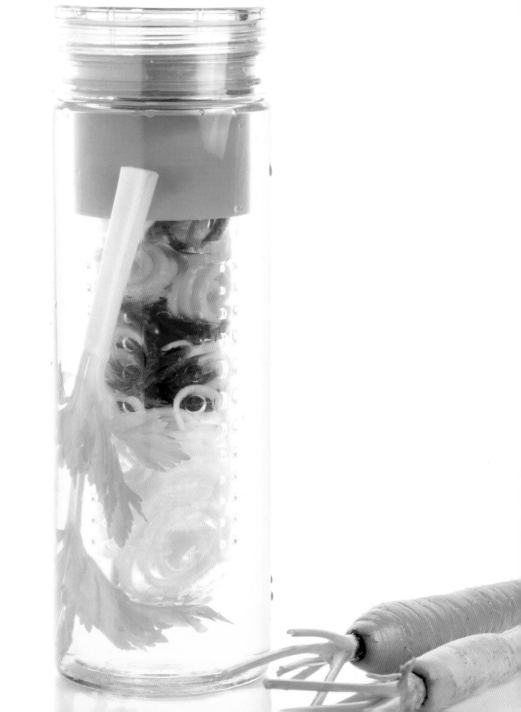

Rainbow Carrots and Celery

SERVINGS: 6–8
PREP TIME: 10 MINUTES
INFUSING TIME: 3–4 HOURS

Ingredients:

1 small bunch rainbow carrots,
   scrubbed and sliced
1 small cucumber, sliced
2 celery sticks
1 tablespoon lemon or lime juice
6–8 cups filtered or spring water

Directions:

Combine carrots, cucumber, and celery in a pitcher and fill with water. Stir in the lemon juice and chill for about 2–4 hours or overnight.

Keep refrigerated and use within 2 days.

TIP
The water will infuse faster if you spiralize the carrots and cucumber.

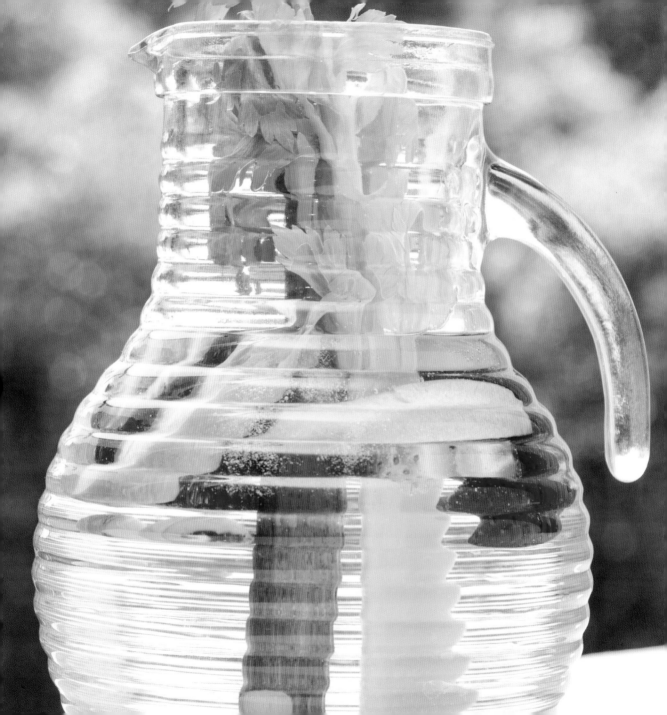

Celery, Rhubarb, Apple, and Strawberry

SERVINGS: 6–8
PREP TIME: 5 MINUTES
INFUSING TIME: OVERNIGHT

Ingredients:

2 sticks celery, cut into 2-inch pieces
2 sticks fresh or frozen rhubarb,* cut into 2-inch pieces
1 Granny Smith apple, cored and sliced
1 cup strawberries, hulled and sliced
6–8 cups filtered or spring water
Ice cubes, to serve

Directions:

Combine all ingredients in pitcher. Fill the pitcher with spring water and refrigerate overnight.

You may refill with water 2–3 times. Serve chilled and use within 2 days.

TIP
*If rhubarb is not available, substitute with fresh or frozen cranberries.

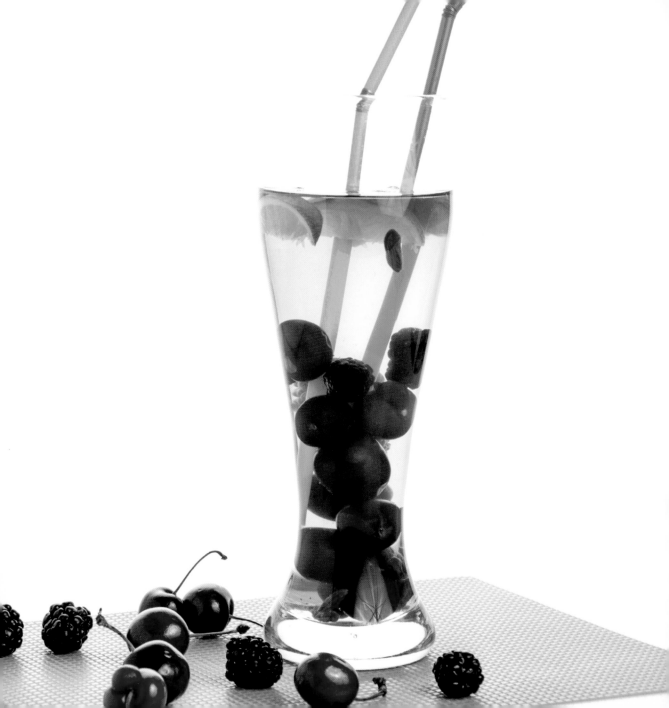

Cherry, Blackberry, and Goji Berry

SERVINGS: 6–8
PREP TIME: 10 MINUTES
INFUSING TIME: 3–4 HOURS

Ingredients:

½ cup fresh or frozen cherries,
   pitted
½ cup blackberries
2–3 tablespoons dried goji berries
2–3 lime slices
6–8 cups filtered or spring water

Directions:

Combine all ingredients in a pitcher or a large jar and refrigerate for 3–4 hours or overnight to allow the flavors to infuse the water. Refill up to 2 times with water and use within 2 days.

TIP
Add a vanilla pod or a few mahlab seeds to further enhance the taste.

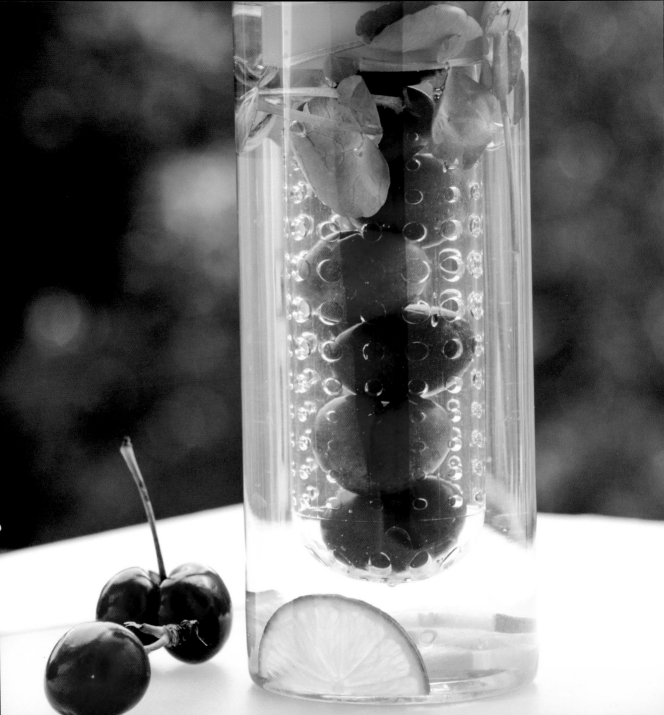

Cherry, Lime, and Watercress

SERVINGS: 4–6
PREP TIME: 10 MINUTES
INFUSING TIME: 3–4 HOURS

Ingredients:

1 cup fresh or frozen cherries,
   pitted
1 handful watercress★
1 handful radish sprouts (optional)
1 lime, sliced
4–6 cups filtered or spring water

Directions:

Place all ingredients in a jar and fill with spring water; refrigerate for 3–4 hours.

Serve chilled and use within 2 days.

TIP
★Substitute watercress with arugula.

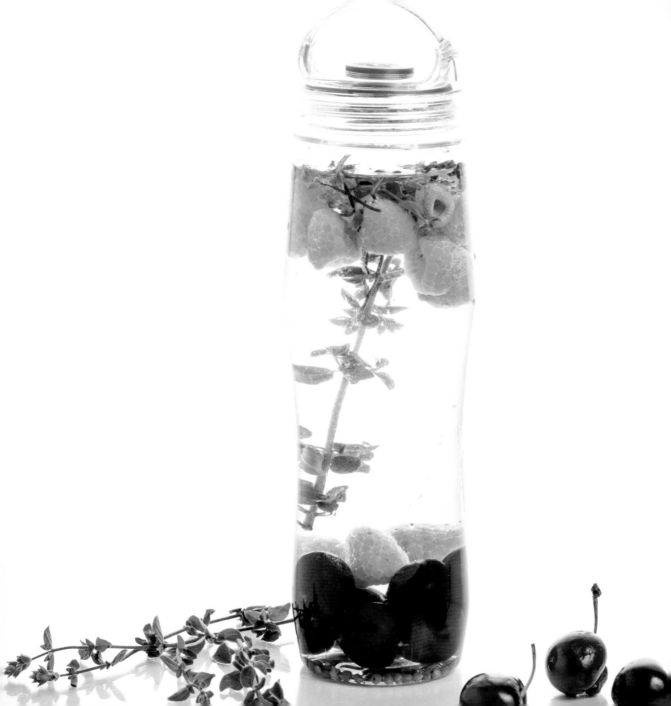

Cherry, Raspberry, and Oregano

SERVINGS: 4–6
PREP TIME: 10 MINUTES
INFUSING TIME: 3–4 HOURS

Ingredients:

1 cup pitted fresh or frozen
   cherries
1 cup raspberries
2 small sprigs fresh oregano*
Sweetener of choice, to taste
6–8 cups filtered or spring water

Directions:

In a large jar, combine cherries, raspberries, and oregano. Add sweetener, if using, and stir. Fill the jar with water and chill for 3–4 hours.

Use within 2 days.

TIP
*Substitute oregano with your favorite fresh herb.

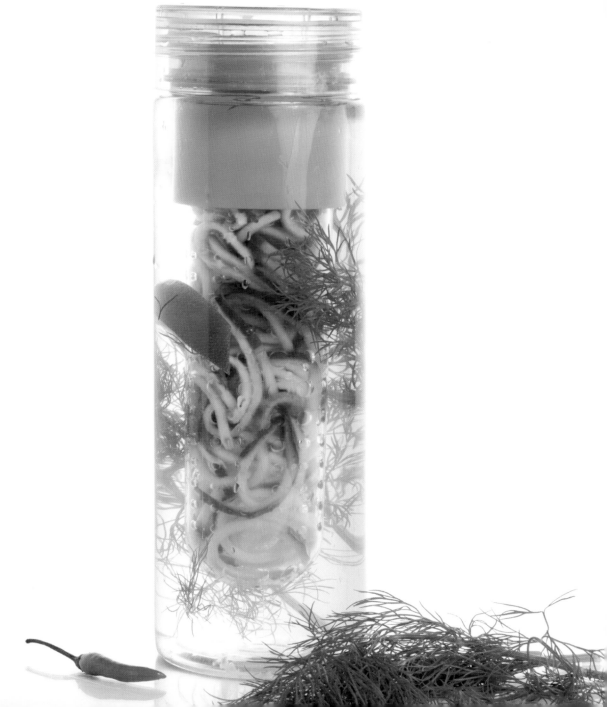

Cucumber, Dill, Garlic, and Lime

SERVINGS: 6–8
PREP TIME: 10 MINUTES
INFUSING TIME: 3–4 HOURS

Ingredients:

2 small cucumbers, thinly sliced
1–2 sprigs fresh dill
1 small garlic clove, cut in half
   lengthwise
1 small green chili pepper, seeded
   (optional)
1 lime, thinly sliced
6–8 cups filtered or spring water

Directions:

Place all ingredients in a pitcher or a large jar; fill with water and refrigerate overnight. Use within 2 days.

TIP
Add ½ thinly sliced fennel and substitute dill with fennel tops.

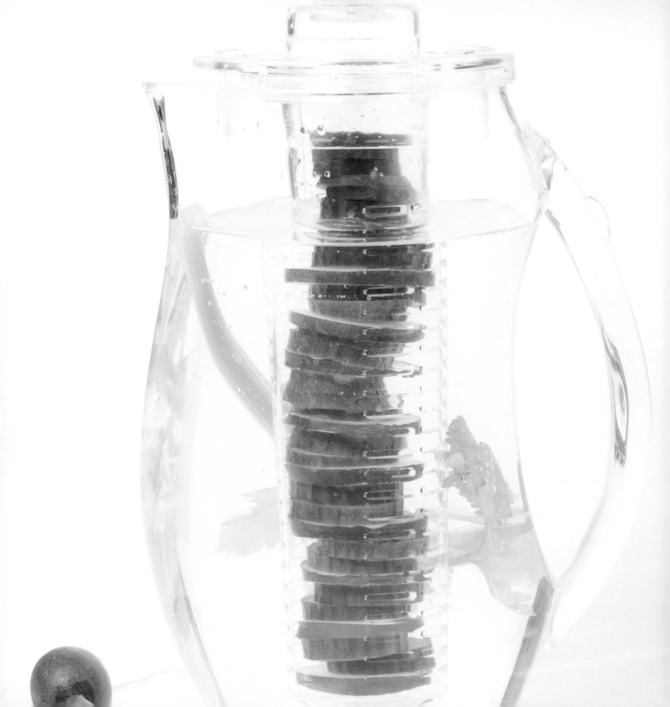

Cucumber, Radish, and Celery

SERVINGS: **6–8**
PREP TIME: **10** MINUTES
INFUSING TIME: OVERNIGHT

Ingredients:

2 cucumbers,★ thinly sliced
½ cup radishes, trimmed and
    thinly sliced
2 celery sticks, cut into 2-inch
    pieces
1 handful parsley (optional)
6–8 cups filtered or spring water

Directions:

Add cucumbers, radishes, celery, and parsley, if using, to a pitcher; fill and refrigerate overnight. You may refill with water 2–3 times. Keep refrigerated and use within 2 days.

TIP
★Use zucchini instead of cucumbers.

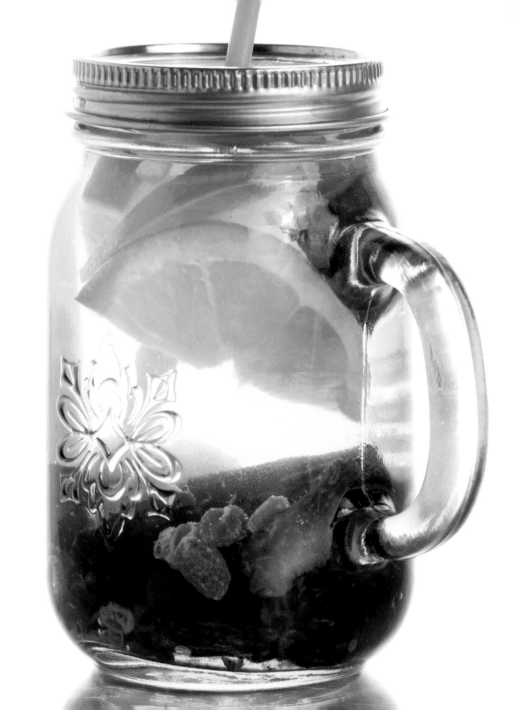
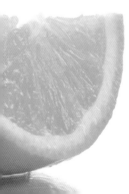

Dried Fruit and Orange

SERVINGS: **6–8**
PREP TIME: **10** MINUTES
INFUSING TIME: OVERNIGHT

Ingredients:

5–6 prunes★
3 tablespoons raisins, sultanas,
    or currants)★
1 orange, sliced
1 cinnamon stick
3–4 whole cloves
1–2 pods star anise
6–8 cups filtered or spring water

Directions:

Combine all ingredients in a large jar or a pitcher and add water. Let infuse overnight. Slice the cactus leaf and rinse multiple times to remove the gelatinous liquid; add to the pitcher together with the oregano, cinnamon bark, and honey.

Use within 2 days.

TIP
★Substitute prunes with dried apricots and raisins with dried cranberries.

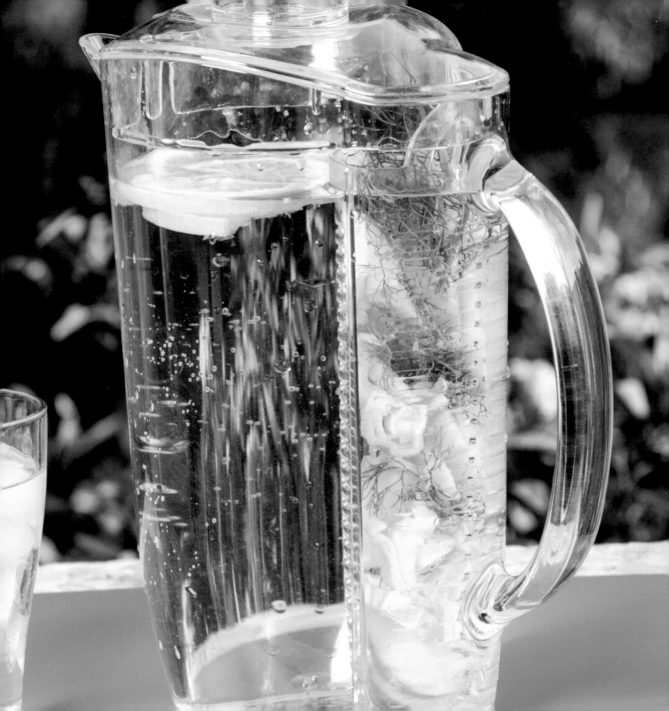

Fennel, Chayote, and Lemon

SERVINGS: 6–8
PREP TIME: 10 MINUTES
INFUSING TIME: 3–4 HOURS, PREFERABLY OVERNIGHT

Ingredients:

1 fennel bulb, trimmed and thinly
   sliced
1 handful fennel tops
1 chayote,* trimmed and thinly
   sliced
1 small lemon, thinly sliced
6–8 cups filtered or spring water

Directions:

Add fennel, fennel tops, chayote, and lemon to a pitcher and fill with water. Chill overnight or a minimum of 3–4 hours to allow the flavors to fully infuse the water. Serve chilled and, if you wish, refill with water 2–3 times. Use within 2 days.

TIP
*Substitute chayote with cucumber or zucchini.

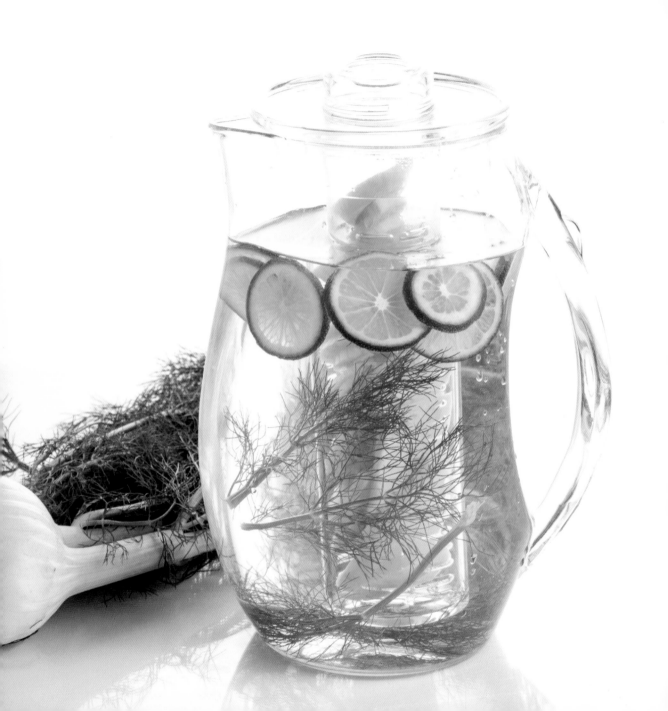

Fennel, Kohlrabi, and Lime

SERVINGS: **4–6**
PREP TIME: **10** MINUTES
INFUSING TIME: **3–4** HOURS

Ingredients:

1 fennel bulb, trimmed and thinly
   sliced
1 handful fennel tops
1 kohlrabi bulb,★ peeled, trimmed,
   and thinly sliced or spiralized
1 lime, thinly sliced
6–8 cups filtered or spring water
Ice cubes, to serve

Directions:

Place all ingredients in a pitcher and fill with water; refrigerate overnight and serve chilled.

You may refill with water 2–3 times.
Keep refrigerated and use within 2 days.

TIP
★Substitute kohlrabi with broccoli stems.

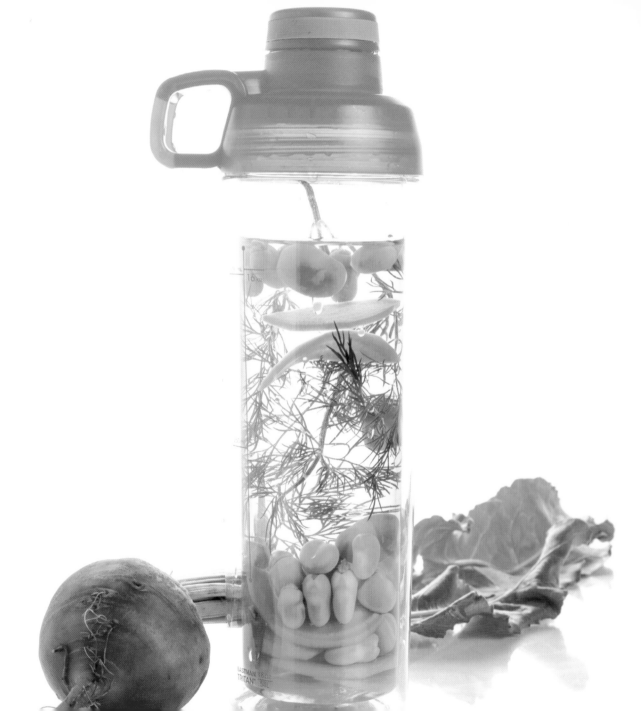

Golden Beet, Fava Beans, and Dill

SERVINGS: 4–6
PREP TIME: 10 MINUTES
INFUSING TIME: OVERNIGHT

Ingredients:

1 golden beet, trimmed, peeled,
   and thinly sliced
½ cup fresh fava beans,* shelled
   and peeled
2–3 dill sprigs
2–3 lemon slices
4–6 cups filtered or spring water
Ice cubes, to serve

Directions:

Combine all ingredients in pitcher. Fill the pitcher with spring water and refrigerate overnight to allow the flavors to fully infuse the water. Serve chilled and use within 2 days.

TIP
*Use young, tender fava beans; if not available, substitute with shelled fresh lima beans or fresh shelled garden peas.

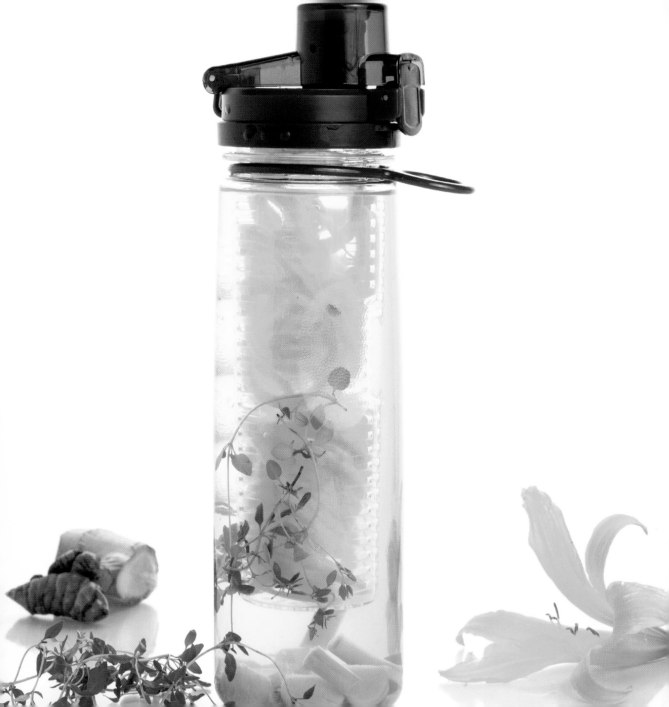

Golden Beet, Turmeric, and Ginger

SERVINGS: 6–8
PREP TIME: 10 MINUTES
INFUSING TIME: OVERNIGHT

Ingredients:

1 golden beet, trimmed, peeled,
and thinly sliced or spiralized
1 (1-inch) piece fresh ginger,
peeled and thinly sliced
1 (2-inch) piece fresh turmeric,
peeled and thinly sliced
1 stalk fresh lemongrass,* tender
part only
A few sprigs fresh thyme or
marjoram
6–8 cups filtered or spring water
Ice cubes, to serve

Directions:

Add beet, ginger, turmeric, lemongrass, and thyme to a pitcher or large jar and fill with water; refrigerate overnight and use within 2 days.

TIP
*Substitute lemongrass with 2–3 shredded sprigs lemon verbena.

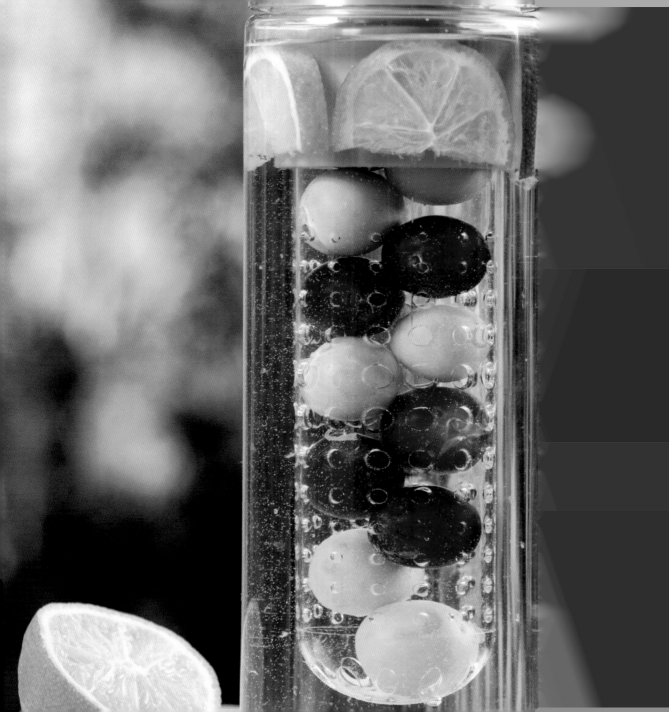

Golden Berries, Red Grapes, and Lime

SERVINGS: **4–6**
PREP TIME: **10** MINUTES
INFUSING TIME: OVERNIGHT

Ingredients:

⅓ cup fresh golden berries,★ halved
⅓ cup seedless red grapes, halved
½ lime, sliced
Sweetener of choice, to taste,
　　optional
4–6 cups filtered or spring water

Directions:

Add golden berries, grapes, and lime to a pitcher and fill with water; refrigerate overnight.

You may refill with water 2–3 times. Keep refrigerated and use within 2 days.

TIP
★If golden berries are not available, use green grapes and add fresh basil leaves.

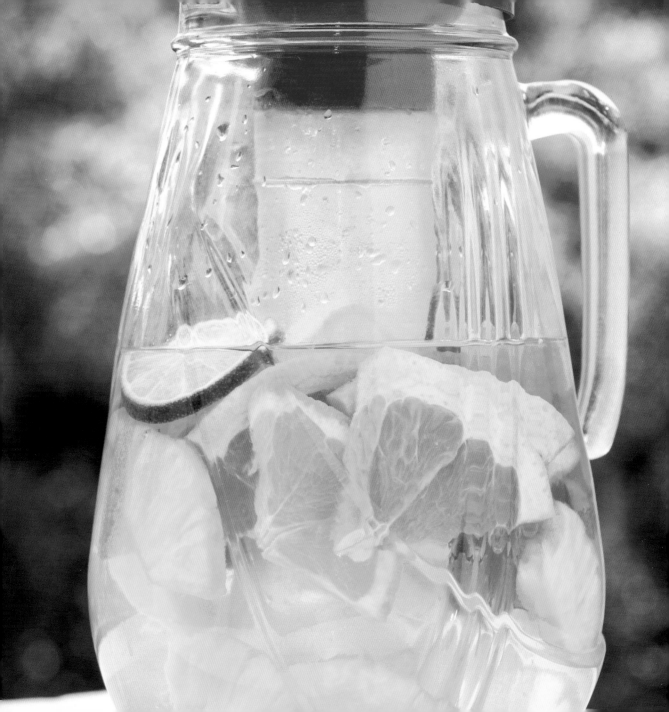

Grapefruit, Orange, Pineapple, and Lime

SERVINGS: 6–8
PREP TIME: 10 MINUTES
INFUSING TIME: 2 HOURS

Ingredients:

½ grapefruit, sliced
1 orange, sliced
½ cup pineapple slices
1 lime, sliced
6–8 cups filtered or spring water
Ice cubes, to serve

Directions:

Add grapefruit, orange, pineapple, and lime slices to a pitcher and fill with water. Chill for about 2 hours and serve over ice.

You may refill with water a few times. Use within 2 days.

TIP
Add ½ to 1 teaspoon orange blossom water.

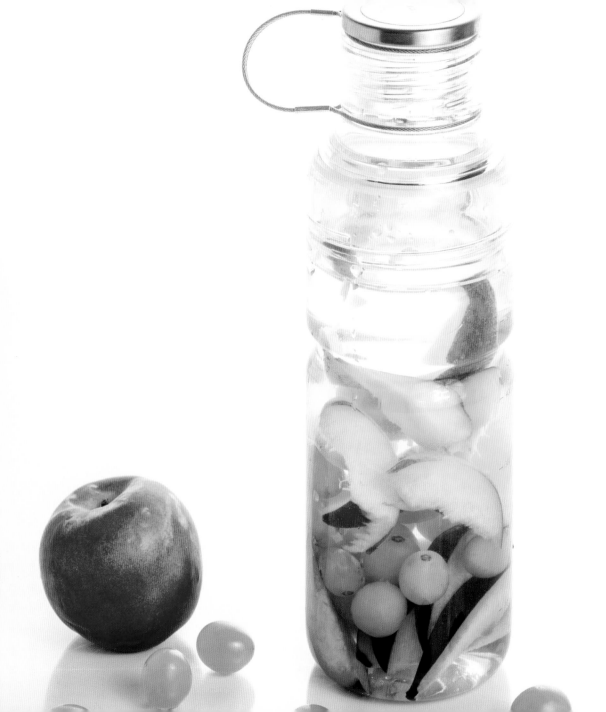

Grapes, Peaches, and Plums

SERVINGS: 4
PREP TIME: 10 MINUTES
INFUSING TIME: 3–4 HOURS

Ingredients:

½ cup seedless green grapes, halved
1 peach, pitted and sliced
2 plums, pitted and sliced
1 (2-inch) piece lemon peel
1 sprig fresh lemon (Thai) basil,
   optional
3–4 cups filtered or spring water
1 teaspoon lemon or lime juice
Ice cubes, to serve

Directions:

Add grapes, peach and plum slices, lemon peel, and basil to an infuser water bottle.

Fill the bottle with water and refrigerate for 3–4 hours or overnight before serving. Refill with water 2–3 times and use within 2 days.

TIP
Add a pinch of ground black pepper or a few crushed peppercorns.

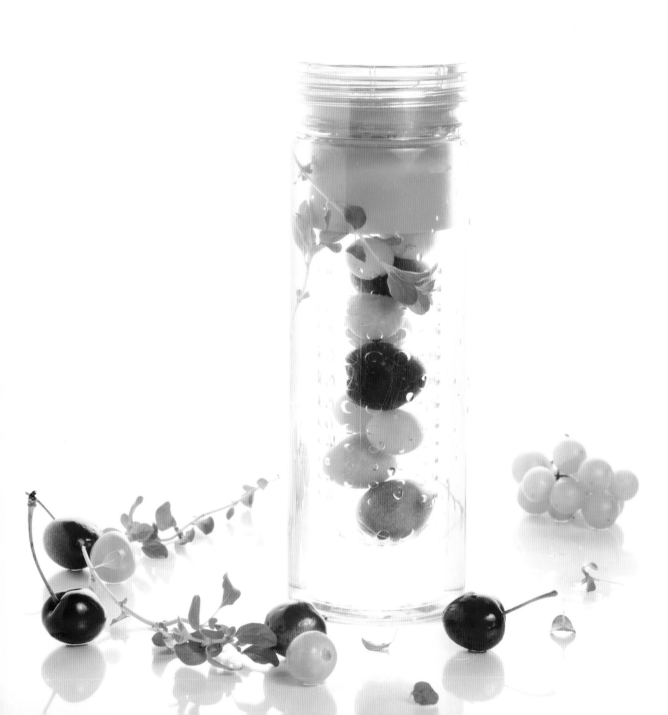

Green Grapes, Cherries, and Golden Berries

SERVINGS: 3–4
PREP TIME: 10 MINUTES
INFUSING TIME: 3–4 HOURS

Ingredients:

⅓ cup seedless green grapes, halved
⅓ cup cherries,★ pitted
⅓ cup golden berries,★ halved
1 small sprig fresh oregano
Sweetener of choice, to taste
6–8 cups filtered or spring water
Ice cubes, to serve

Directions:

Combine grapes, cherries, and golden berries in an infuser water bottle or a jar. Add oregano and sweetener, if using. Fill the bottle with spring water and refrigerate for 3–4 hours or overnight.

Refill with water 2–3 times and use within 2 days.

TIP
★Substitute cherries and golden berries with seedless red grapes.

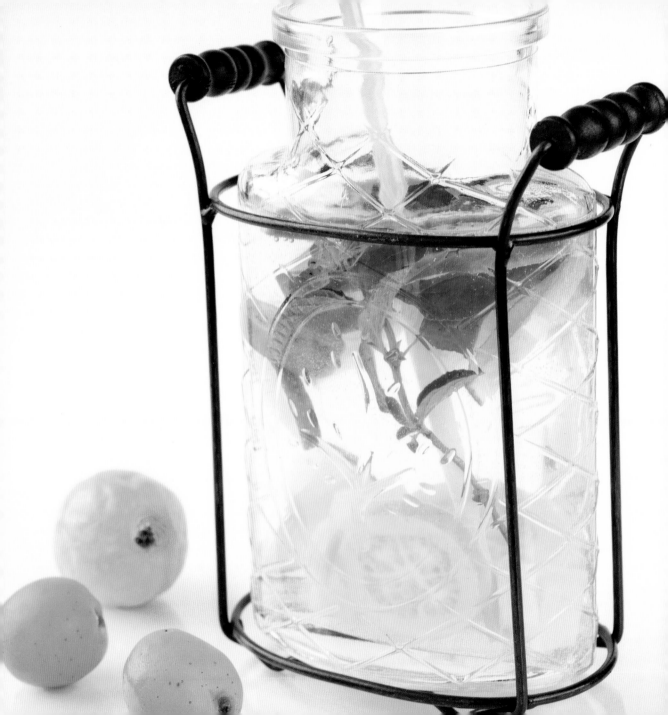

Guava, Lime, and Cactus Leaf

SERVINGS: **4–6**
PREP TIME: **10** MINUTES
INFUSING TIME: **3–4** HOURS

Ingredients:

3–4 tejocotes,* sliced
3 guavas,** sliced
1 lime, sliced
2 (1½–2 inch) pieces peeled sugar
 cane
1 (2-inch) piece fresh cactus leaf,
 spines removed and thinly sliced
1 sprig fresh oregano
1 (1½-inch) piece cinnamon bark
1 teaspoon raw honey or other
 sweetener of choice, optional
4–6 cups filtered or spring water
Ice cubes, to serve

Directions:

Slice the tejocotes, guavas, lime, and sugar cane into ¼-inch thick slices and place in a large jar.

Slice the cactus leaf and rinse multiple times to remove the gelatinous liquid; add to the pitcher together with the oregano, cinnamon bark, and honey.

Fill the pitcher with spring water and refrigerate for 3–4 hours to allow the flavors to infuse the water. You may refill with water 2–3 times. Use within 2 days.

TIP
*Fresh tejocotes (also called hawthorn apples or Mexican apples) are in season from October to December and are used in ponche, a Mexican fruit punch traditionally served at Christmas. Substitute with kumquats or apricots, if not available.
**Substitute guavas with peeled and sliced quince or pear.

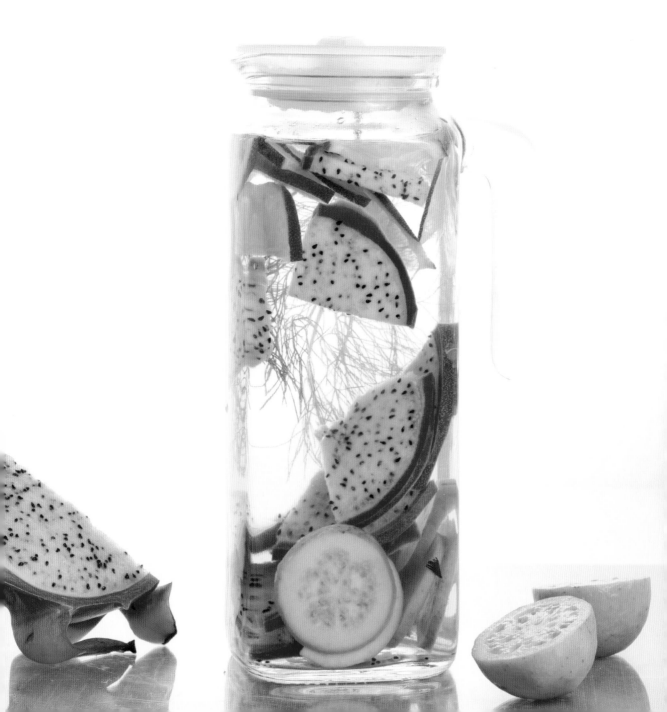

Guava, Lime, Dragon Fruit, and Fennel Tops

SERVINGS: **4–6**
PREP TIME: **10** MINUTES
INFUSING TIME: **3–4** HOURS

Ingredients:

3–4 guavas,★ sliced
1 lime, sliced
½ dragon fruit,★ trimmed and sliced
1 small fennel frond★
Sweetener of choice, to taste,
    optional
4–6 cups filtered or spring water

Directions:

Place sliced guavas, lime, dragon fruit, and fennel in a pitcher or a large jar.

Fill the pitcher with spring water, add sweetener, if using, and stir. Refrigerate for 3–4 hours or overnight.

Refill with water 2–3 times and use within 2 days.

TIP
★Substitute guavas with cored and sliced pear and the dragon fruit with kiwi. Add a few leaves fresh tarragon instead of the fennel tops.

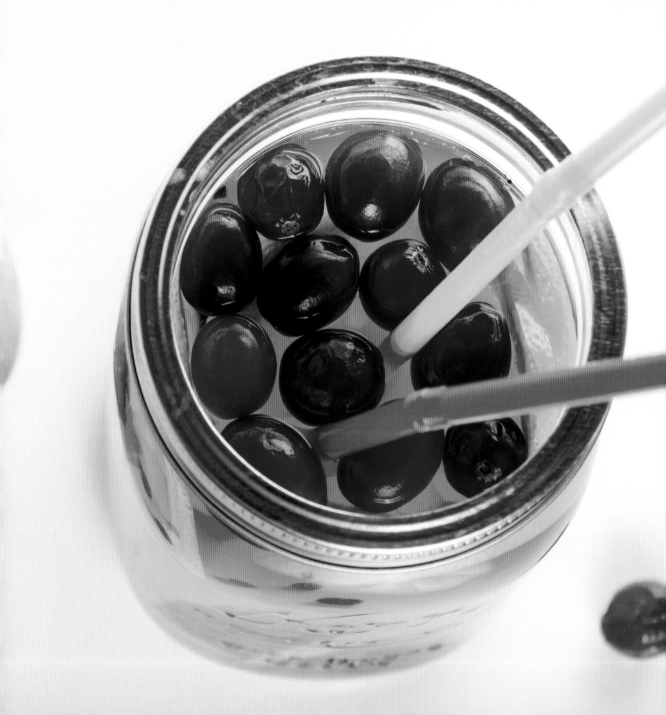

Hibiscus, Pear, Ginger, and Cranberries

Servings: 4–6
Prep Time: 10 minutes
Infusing Time: ovenight

Ingredients:

3–4 dried hibiscus flowers
1 pear, cored and sliced
2–3 lemon slices
1 knob (about 1½-inch) fresh
   ginger, peeled and sliced
⅓ cup fresh or frozen cranberries
½ teaspoon fennel seeds,* optional
Sweetener of choice, to taste,
   optional
4–6 cups filtered or spring water

Directions:

In a large jar, combine dried hibiscus flowers, pear, lemon and ginger slices, cranberries, and fennel seeds.

Fill the jar with water and stir in sweetener, if using. Let the water infuse overnight in the fridge.

If desired, refill with water and use within 2–3 days.

TIP
*Substitute fennel seeds with 1–2 pods of star anise or ½ teaspoon aniseed.

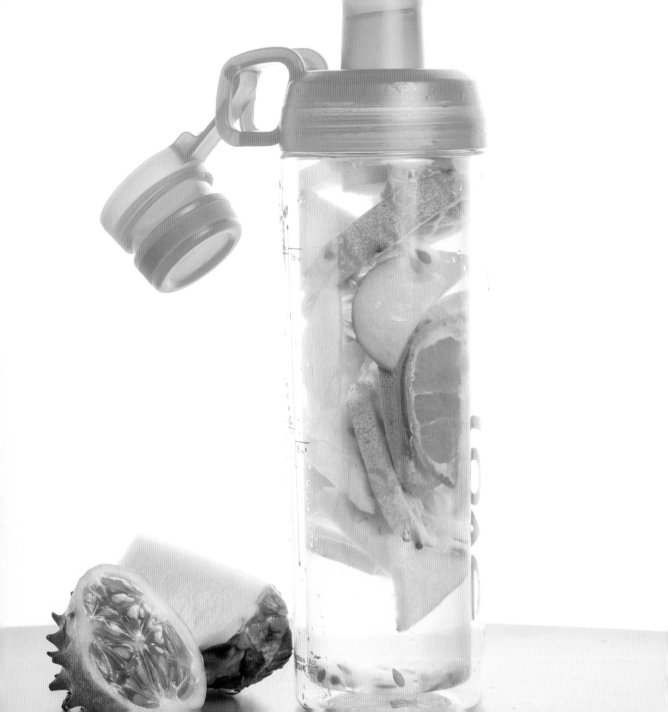

Horned Melon (Kiwano), Pineapple, Chayote, and Mandarin Orange

SERVINGS: 6–8
PREP TIME: 10 MINUTES
INFUSING TIME: 3–4 HOURS

Ingredients:

1 kiwano,⋆ trimmed and sliced
½ cup sliced pineapple
1 chayote,⋆ trimmed and sliced
1 mandarin orange, sliced
6–8 cups filtered or spring water
Ice cubes, to serve

Directions:

Place kiwano, pineapple, chayote, and mandarin orange slices in a pitcher; fill with water and refrigerate for 3–4 hours.

Serve over ice and use within 2 days.

TIP
⋆Kiwano and chayote may be substituted with cucumber or melon.

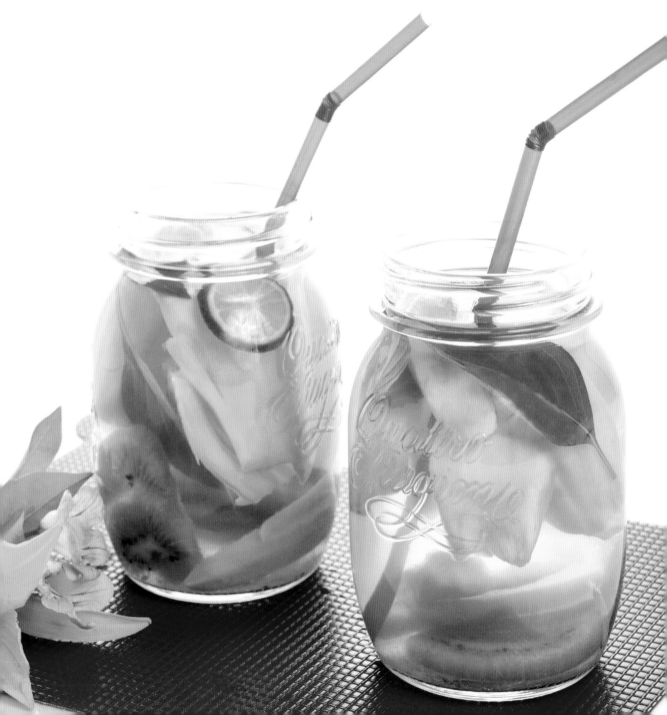

Jackfruit, Kiwi, and Key Lime

SERVINGS: 4–6
PREP TIME: 10 MINUTES
INFUSING TIME: OVERNIGHT

Ingredients:

⅓ cup ripe jackfruit,★ cut into
    strips
2 kiwis, peeled and sliced
2–3 key limes, sliced thinly
1–2 sprigs Thai basil
4–6 cups filtered or spring water
Ice cubes

Directions:

In a large jar, combine jackfruit, kiwi, key limes, and basil. Fill with water and place in the fridge to infuse overnight.

Serve over ice and use within 2 days.

TIP
★Substitute jackfruit with mango.

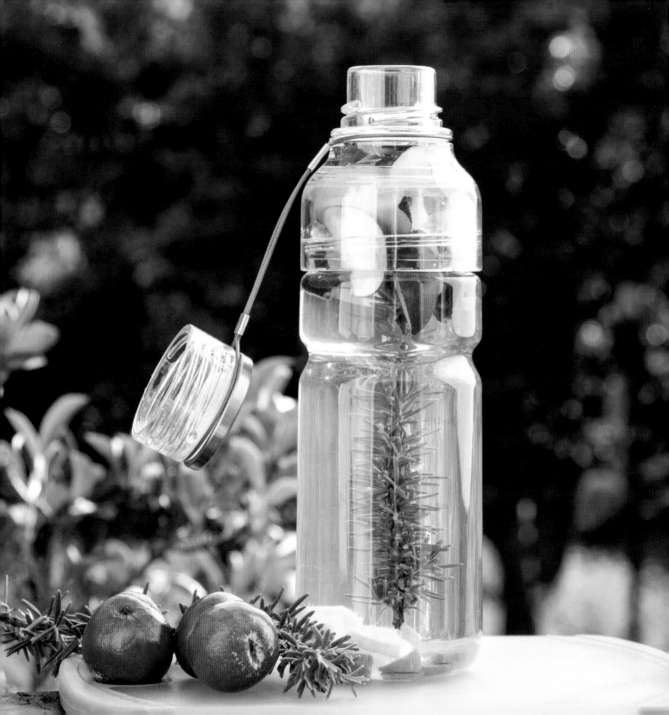

Jujube, Rosemary, Ginger, and Turmeric

SERVINGS: **4–6**
PREP TIME: **10** MINUTES
INFUSING TIME: **3–4** HOURS

Ingredients:

3–4 fresh jujubes,★ sliced
1 sprig fresh rosemary
1 (1-inch) piece fresh ginger, peeled and sliced
1 (2-inch) piece fresh turmeric, peeled and sliced
1–2 limes, sliced
3–4 cups filtered or spring water

Directions:

Place sliced jujube, rosemary, ginger, turmeric, and lime into an infuser water bottle or a jar.

Pour the water into the jar; cover with a lid and refrigerate for at least two hours or overnight for the best flavor. Drink within 2 days.

TIP
★Jujube fruit is also known as red date, Chinese date, Korean date, or Indian date. You may substitute fresh jujubes with plums or apples.

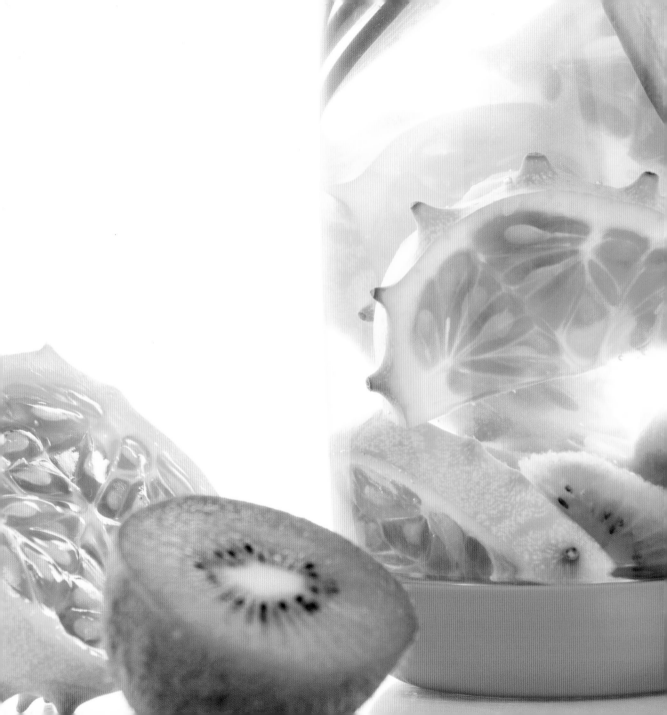

Kiwano, Cucumber, and Kiwi

SERVINGS: 4–6
PREP TIME: 10 MINUTES
INFUSING TIME: 3–4 HOURS

Ingredients:

1 kiwano,* trimmed and sliced
1 cucumber, sliced
2 kiwis, peeled and sliced
A few fresh chives
4–6 cups filtered or spring water
Ice cubes, to serve

Directions:

Combine the kiwano, cucumber, kiwis, and chives in a pitcher. Fill the pitcher with spring water and refrigerate for 3–4 hours to allow the flavors to infuse the water. You may refill with water 2–3 times. Use within 2 days.

TIP
*If kiwano (horned melon) is not available, use additional kiwi and/or cucumber.

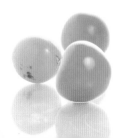
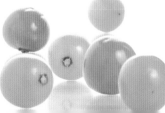
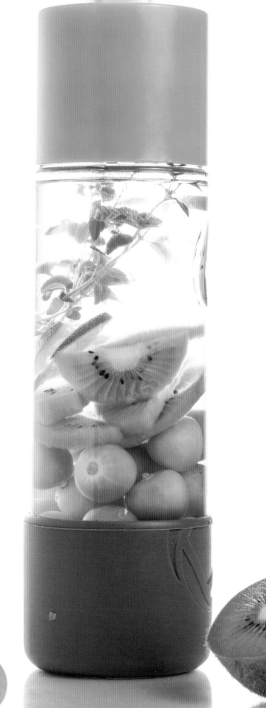

Kiwi, Golden Berries, Green Grapes, and Thyme

SERVINGS: **4–6**
PREP TIME: **10** MINUTES
INFUSING TIME: **4** HOURS

Ingredients:

2 kiwis, peeled and sliced
⅓ cup fresh golden berries,* halved
⅓ cup seedless green grapes, halved
1–2 sprigs fresh thyme or
    marjoram
Sweetener of choice, to taste,
    optional
4–6 cups filtered or spring water
Ice cubes, to serve

Directions:

In a jar or infuser water bottle, combine kiwi, golden berries, grapes, and thyme.

Fill water and refrigerate for about 4 hours or overnight.

Serve chilled and use within 2 days.

TIP
*Golden berries (also known as Cape gooseberries) can be substituted with tomatillos or gooseberries.

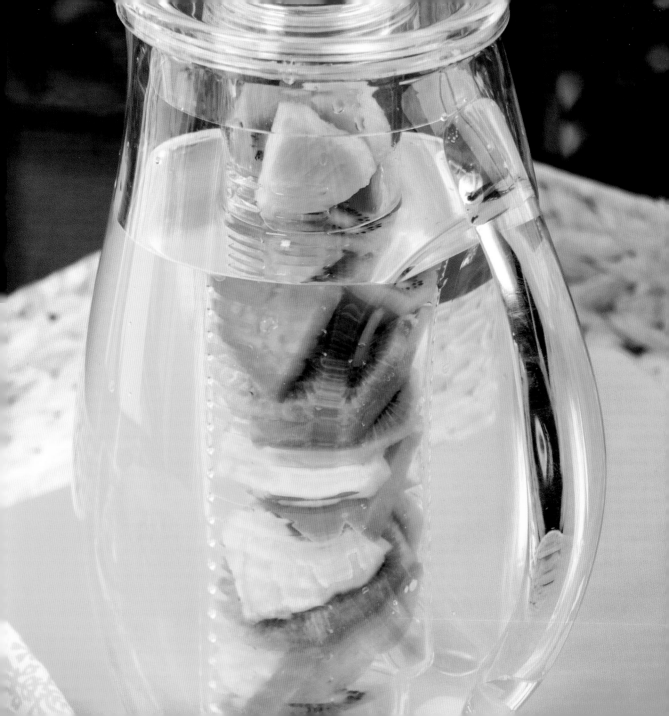

Kiwi, Papaya, and Pineapple

SERVINGS: 6–8
PREP TIME: 10 MINUTES
INFUSING TIME: 3–4 HOURS

Ingredients:

2 kiwis, peeled and sliced
⅔ cup peeled and sliced pineapple
⅔ cup peeled and sliced papaya
A pinch of saffron threads★
6–8 cups filtered or spring water
Ice cubes, to serve

Directions:

Add all ingredients to a pitcher and fill with water; chill for 3–4 hours or overnight before serving.

Refill with water and use within 2–3 days.

TIP
★Substitute saffron with 1-inch knob fresh turmeric.

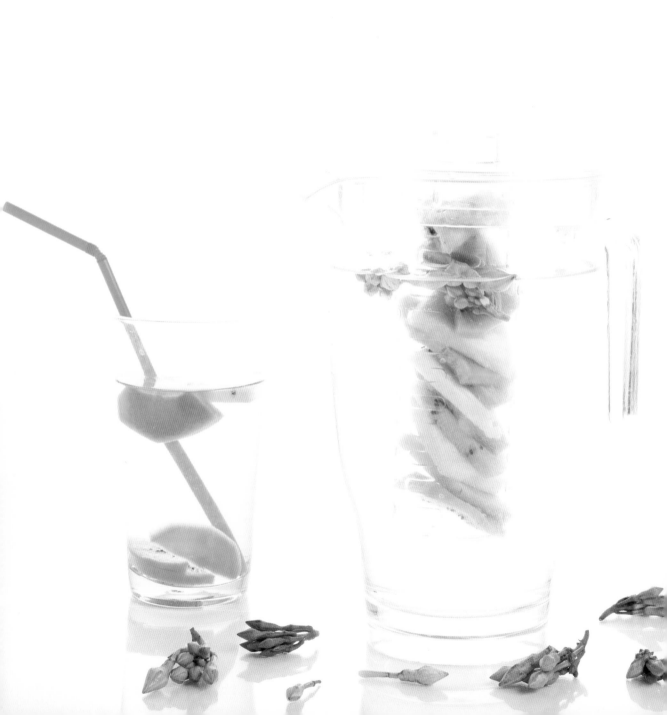

Kiwi, Persimmon, Pineapple, and Loroco Flowers

SERVINGS: 6–8
PREP TIME: 10 MINUTES
INFUSING TIME: 3–4 HOURS

Ingredients:

2 kiwis, peeled and sliced
1 Fuyu persimmon, trimmed
   and sliced
½ cup sliced pineapple
1–2 small clusters loroco flower
   buds★
1–2 lime slices
6–8 cups filtered or spring water

Directions:

Add all ingredients to a pitcher and fill with water; refrigerate overnight and serve chilled.

Use within 2 days.

TIP
★Loroco is a woody vine native to South America. The flower buds have a unique flavor and are used as an herb. It is available in some farmer's markets, but if not, substitute with a small handful of cilantro.

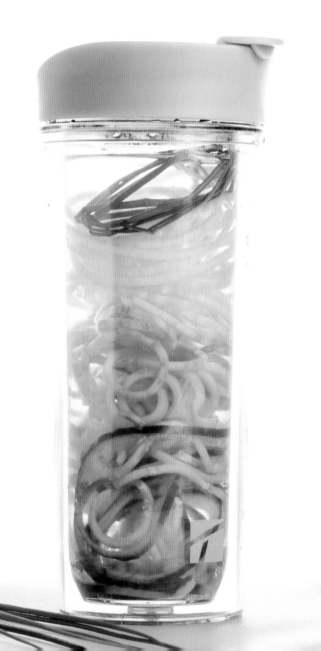

Korean Radish, Broccoli Stem, Cucumber, and Chives

SERVINGS: 6–8
PREP TIME: 10 MINUTES
INFUSING TIME: 3–4 HOURS

Ingredients:

⅔ cup Korean radish,★ peeled and thinly sliced or spiralized

1 (4-inch piece) broccoli stem, thinly sliced or spiralized

1 small cucumber, trimmed and sliced or spiralized

A few fresh chives

2–3 lime or lemon slices

1 serrano pepper, seeded, optional

6–8 cups filtered or spring water

Directions:

Add the vegetables to a large jar and fill with water; refrigerate for 3–4 hours before serving. Use within 2 days.

TIP
★Substitute Korean radish with Daikon radish.

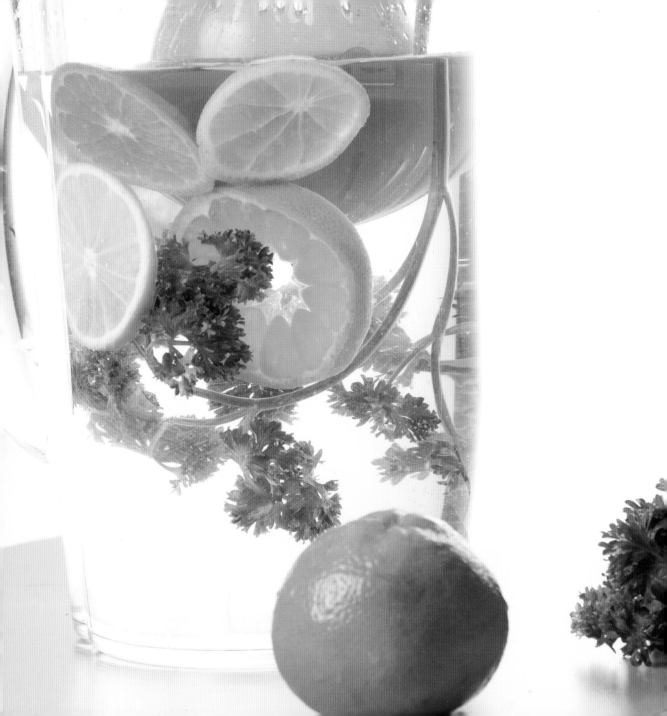

Mandarin Orange, Lime, Parsley, and Lemon

SERVINGS: 6–8
PREP TIME: 10 MINUTES
INFUSING TIME: 2–4 HOURS

Ingredients:

2 mandarin oranges, sliced or
  segmented
1 lime, sliced
½ lemon, sliced
A small handful parsley sprigs
6–8 cups filtered or spring water
Ice cubes, to serve

Directions:

Add mandarin oranges, lime, lemon, and parsley to a pitcher and fill with spring water.

Allow the flavors to infuse in the fridge about 2 hours before serving. Use within 5–6 hours.

TIP
You may vary the flavor by adding any combination of citrus fruit and substituting the parsley with other fresh herbs, such as cilantro or mint.

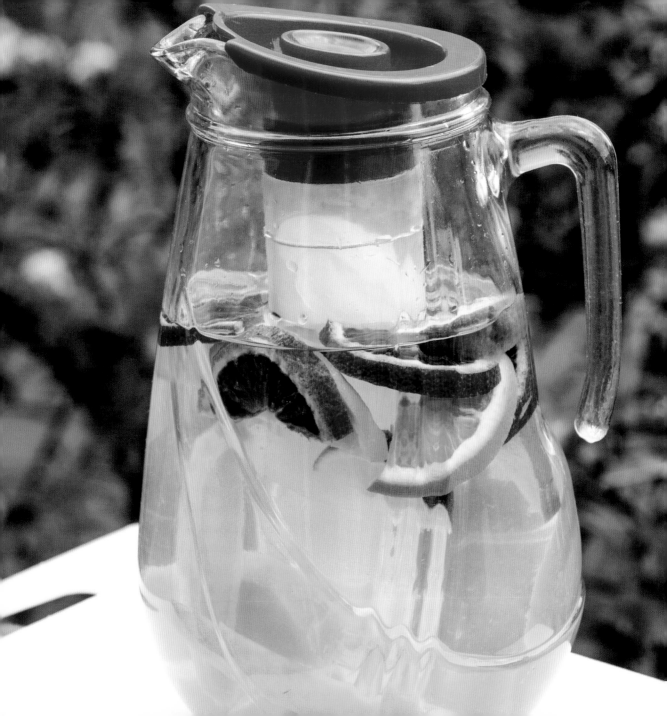

Mango, Blood Orange, and Lime

Servings: 6–8
Prep Time: 10 minutes
Infusing Time: 3–4 hours

Ingredients:

1 mango, pitted, peeled, and sliced
2 blood oranges,* sliced
½ lime, sliced
6–8 cups filtered or spring water
Ice cubes, to serve

Directions:

Place mango, blood oranges, and lime in a pitcher. Fill the pitcher with spring water and refrigerate for 2–3 hours to allow the flavors to infuse the water.

The orange rind will cause a slightly bitter taste, so it is best to use the infused water within 5–6 hours.

TIP
*If blood oranges are not available, use any other citrus fruit.

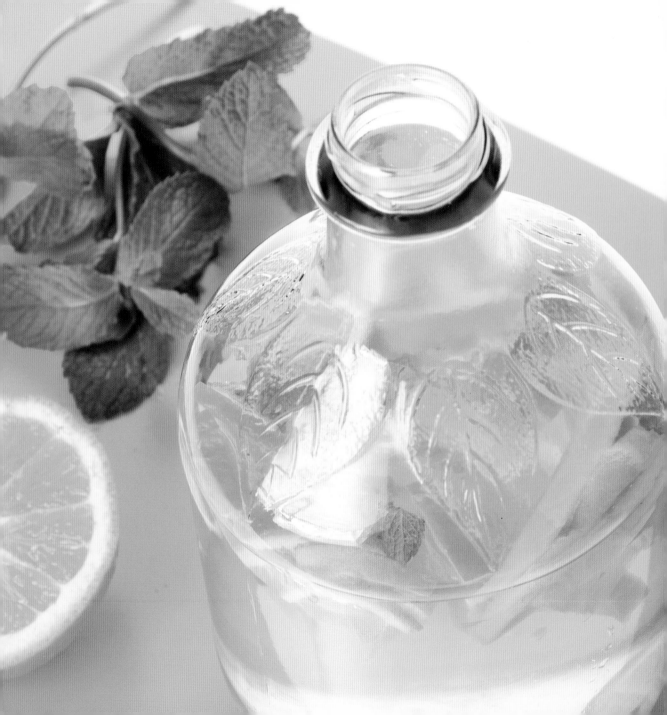

Mango, Lemon, Tangerine, and Pear

SERVINGS: 6–8
PREP TIME: 10 MINUTES
INFUSING TIME: 3–4 HOURS

Ingredients:

1 mango, pitted, peeled, and sliced
½ lemon, thinly sliced
1 tangerine, segmented
1 pear, cored and thinly sliced
2–3 fresh mint* sprigs
6–8 cups filtered or spring water
Ice cubes, to serve

Directions:

In a large jar or a pitcher, combine mango, lemon, tangerine, and pear; add mint and fill with water; chill for 3–4 hours.

Serve chilled and use within 2 days.

TIP
*Substitute mint with other fresh herbs of choice.

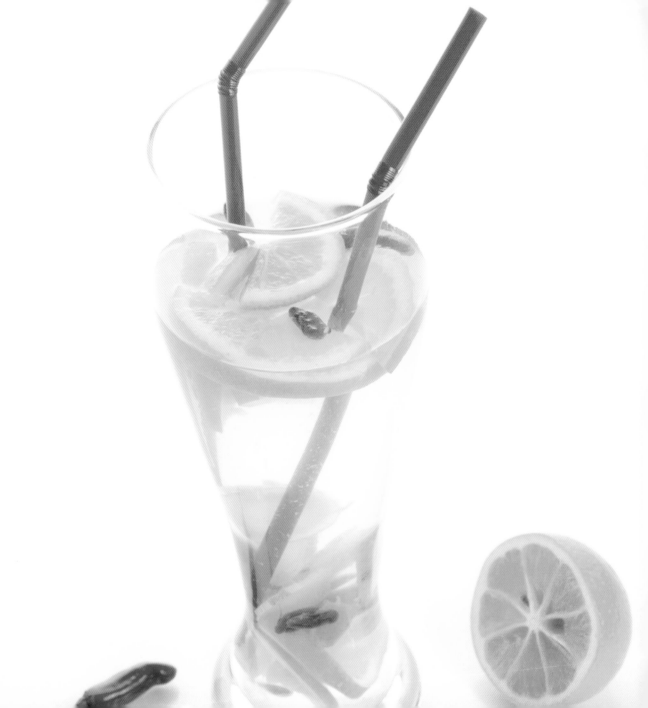

Meyer Lemon, Ginger, Red Chili, and Turmeric

SERVINGS: 6–8
PREP TIME: 10 MINUTES
INFUSING TIME: 2–3 HOURS

Ingredients:

2 Meyer lemons, sliced
1 (1½-inch) piece fresh ginger, peeled and sliced
1 (2-inch) piece fresh turmeric, peeled and sliced
2–3 small red chillies or to taste
2 tablespoons dried goji berries, optional
6–8 cups filtered or spring water
Ice cubes, to serve

Directions:

Add Meyer lemons, ginger, turmeric, red chillies, and goji berries, if using, to a pitcher. Fill with spring water and allow to steep in the fridge for 3–4 hours.

Serve chilled.

TIP
Add additional flavor with a piece of cinnamon bark.

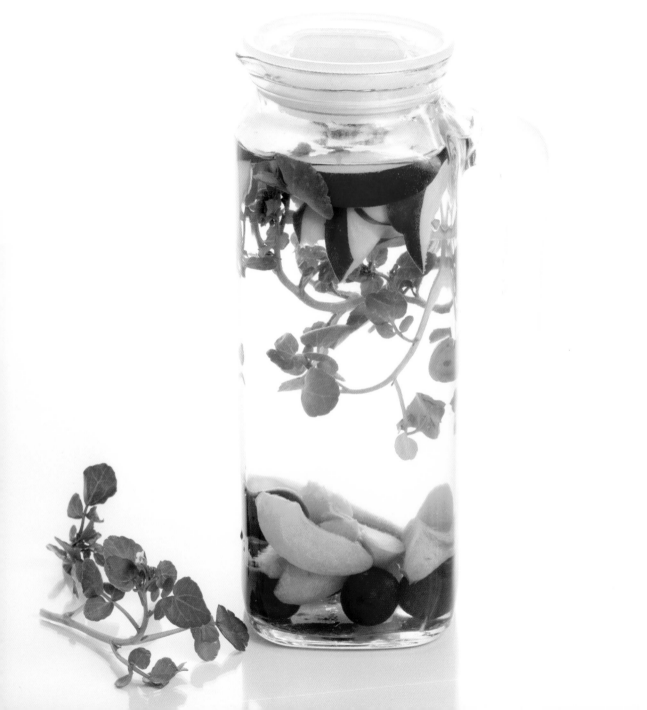

Nectarine, Apricot, Red Grapes, and Watercress

SERVINGS: **4–6**
PREP TIME: **10** MINUTES
INFUSING TIME: **3–4** HOURS

Ingredients:

1 nectarine, pitted and sliced
2 apricots, pitted and sliced
½ cup red grapes, halved
A handful watercress*
4–6 cups filtered or spring water
Ice cubes, to serve

Directions:

Place nectarine, apricots, grapes, and watercress in a large jar or another glass container with a lid and fill with water.

Refrigerate for 3–4 hours to overnight before serving. Use within 24 hours.

TIP
*Substitute watercress with baby arugula.

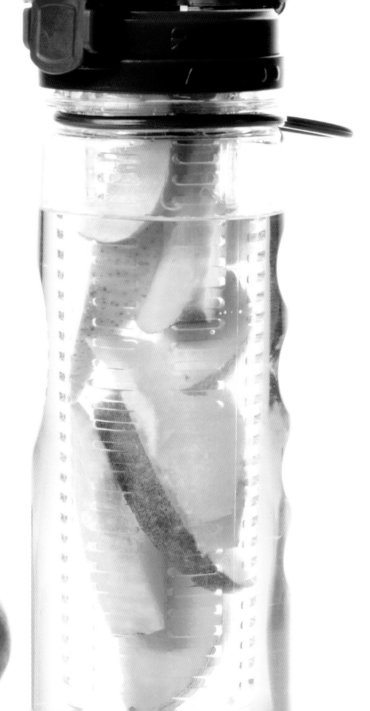

Nectarine, Pear, and Lime

SERVINGS: 3–4
PREP TIME: 10 MINUTES
INFUSING TIME: 3–4 HOURS

Ingredients:

1 nectarine, pitted and sliced
1 pear, cored and sliced
1 lime, sliced
¼ teaspoon dried culinary
    lavender,* optional
3–4 cups filtered or spring water

Directions:

Add nectarine, pear, and lime slices to an infuser water bottle and fill with water.

Allow to steep in the refrigerator for 2–4 hours before serving.

Refill the bottle with water a couple of times and use within 2 days.

TIP
*Lavender has a very strong flavor, so adjust the quantity to your taste.

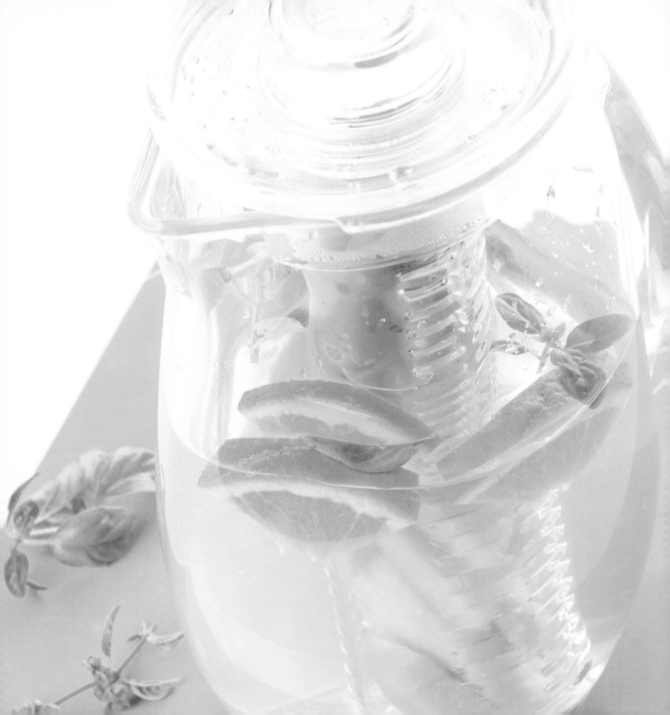

Orange, Cantaloupe, Kumquats, and Basil

SERVINGS: 6–8
PREP TIME: 10 MINUTES
INFUSING TIME: 3–4 HOURS

Ingredients:

1 orange, sliced
1 cup cantaloupe, peeled and diced
   or sliced
⅔ cup kumquats,* quartered and
   seeded
1 (1-inch) piece fresh ginger,
   peeled and sliced, optional
2–3 fresh basil sprigs
6–8 cups filtered or spring water
Ice cubes, to serve

Directions:

In a pitcher or a large glass, add orange, cantaloupe, kumquats, ginger slices, and basil and fill with water.

Allow it to infuse for about 2 hours in the refrigerator before serving.

Serve within 4–6 hours for best taste.

TIP
*Substitute kumquats with mandarin orange segments.

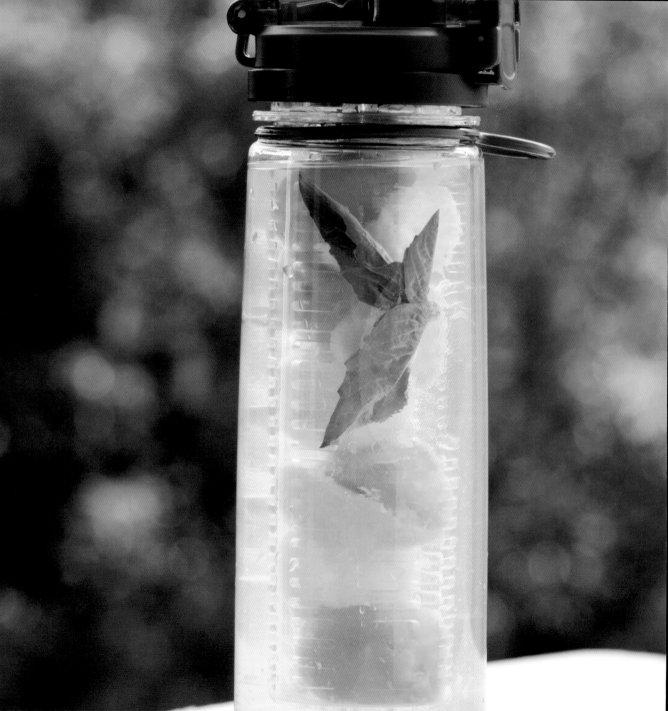

Papaya, Mango, Pineapple, and Thai Basil

SERVINGS: **2–3**
PREP TIME: **10** MINUTES
INFUSING TIME: **2–4** HOURS

Ingredients:

¼ cup papaya slices
¼ cup pineapple slices
¼ cup mango slices
1–2 sprigs Thai basil
1 lime, sliced, optional
2–3 cups filtered or spring water★

Directions:

Add papaya, pineapple, mango, and basil to an infuser water bottle and fill with water.

Chill for 2–4 hours before serving.

You may refill with water 2–3 times. Use within 2 days.

TIP
★Use coconut water for an amazingly refreshing tropical taste.

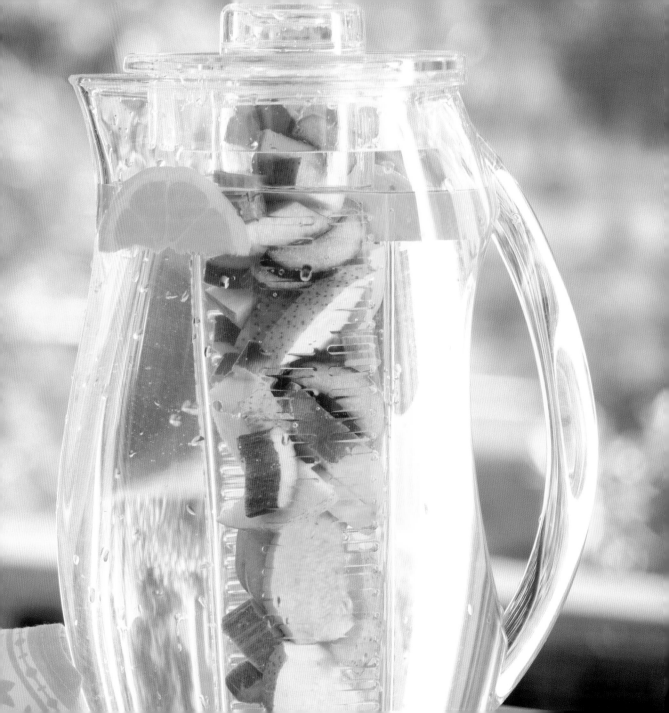

Pear, Apple, Quince, and Rhubarb

SERVINGS: 6–8
PREP TIME: 10 MINUTES
INFUSING TIME: 3–4 HOURS

Ingredients:

1 pear, cored and sliced
1 apple, cored and sliced
1 quince, trimmed, cored,
   and sliced
1 rhubarb stalk, sliced
2–3 lemon slices
6–8 cups filtered or spring water

Directions:

Place the ingredients in a pitcher and fill with water. Chill for about 3–4 hours or overnight before serving.

Refill with water 2–3 times and use within 2 days.

TIP
Spice it up with a few allspice berries or crushed cardamom pods. If quince is not in season, substitute with Asian pear.

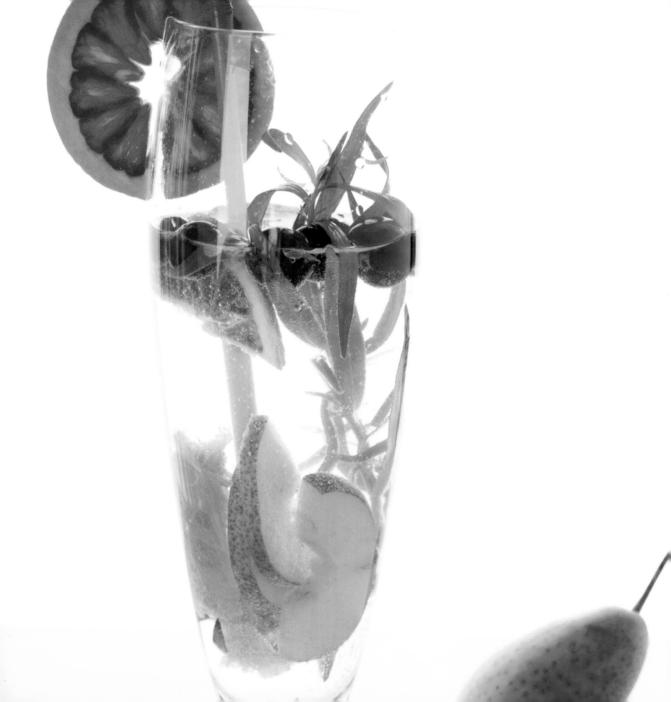

Pear, Cranberry, Blood Orange, and Pink Grapefruit

SERVINGS: **6–8**
PREP TIME: **5** MINUTES
INFUSING TIME: **2–3** HOURS

Ingredients:

2 small pears, cored and sliced
¼ cup fresh or frozen cranberries
½ pink grapefruit, peeled and
   segmented
1 blood orange, sliced
1 small sprig fresh tarragon
6–8 cups filtered or spring water

Directions:

In a pitcher or a large glass jar, combine pears, cranberries, grapefruit segments, orange slices, and tarragon.

Add water and refrigerate for at least 2–3 hours to allow flavors to infuse before serving.

Refill with water 2–3 times and use within 2 days.

TIP
Adding a few green peppercorns will give the water a fresh, crisp taste.

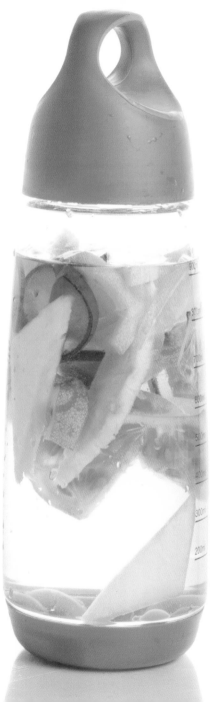
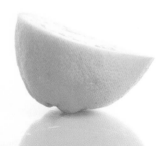

Pineapple, Kiwano, Kumquats, and Aloe Vera

SERVINGS: 4–6
PREP TIME: 5 MINUTES
INFUSING TIME: 2–3 HOURS

Ingredients:

½ cup sliced pineapple
½ kiwano,★ sliced
2–3 kumquats, halved and seeded
1–2 cups aloe vera juice
1 small sprig rosemary
1–2 lemon slices
Sweetener of choice, to taste, optional
3–4 cups filtered or spring water

Directions:

In a water bottle or a glass jar, combine pineapple, kiwano, kumquats, aloe vera juice, rosemary, lemon, and sweetener, if using.

Add water and refrigerate for 3–4 hours to allow flavors to infuse before serving.

Refill with water 2–3 times and use within 2 days.

TIP
★Make sure the kiwano (also called horned melon or African horned cucumber) is fully ripened, with yellow-orange rind and spikes.

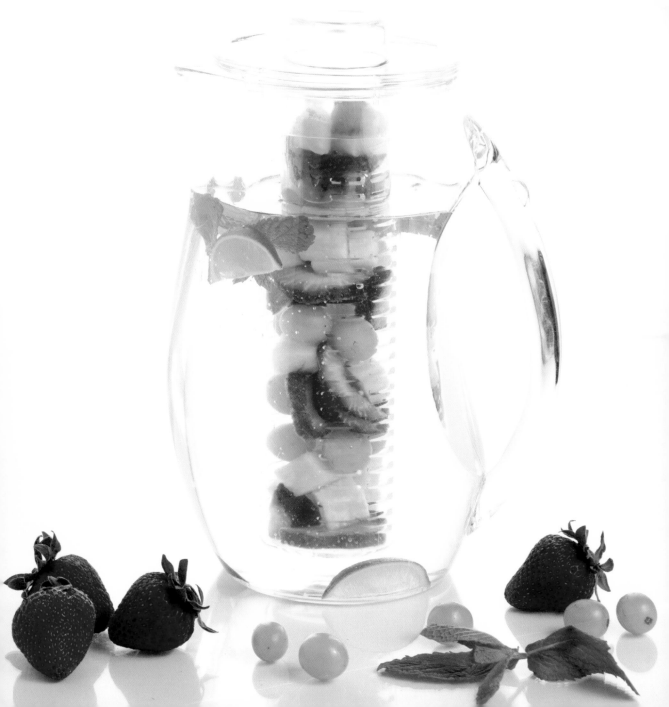

Pineapple, Strawberry, and Grapes

SERVINGS: 6–8
PREP TIME: 10 MINUTES
INFUSING TIME: 3–4 HOURS

Ingredients:

⅔ cup pineapple slices
4–5 strawberries, hulled and sliced
½ cup seedless green grapes, halved
1 lime, thinly sliced
6–8 cups filtered or spring water
Ice cubes, to serve

Directions:

In a pitcher, combine pineapple, strawberry, grapes, and lime and fill with water. Refrigerate for 3–4 hours and serve over ice.

You may refill with water once or twice. Use within 2 days.

TIP
Add 1–2 sprigs fresh mint or another fresh herb, such as basil.

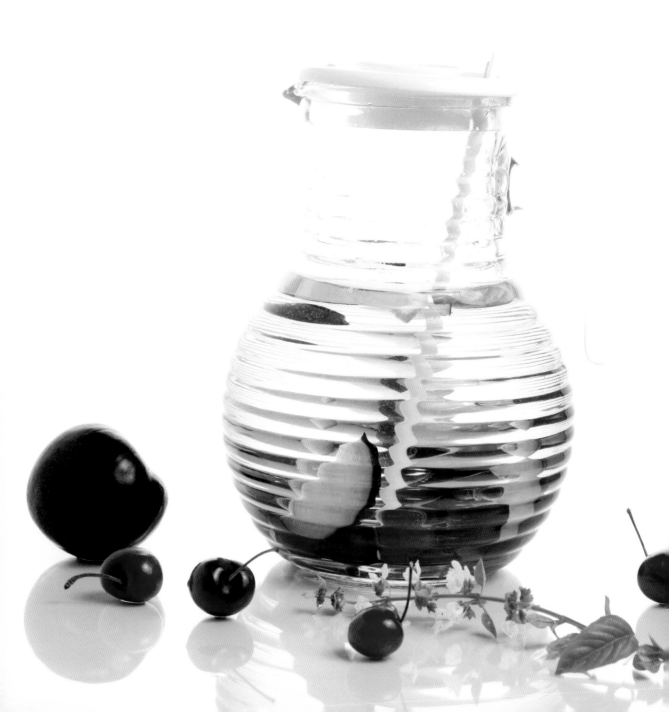

Plum, Cherry, Lemon, and Basil

SERVINGS: **4–6**
PREP TIME: **10** MINUTES
INFUSING TIME: **3–4** HOURS

Ingredients:

2–3 plums, pitted and sliced
1 handful cherries, stemmed
    and pitted
1 lime, thinly sliced
1–2 sprigs fresh basil
3–4 whole mahlab seeds,⋆ optional
4–6 cups filtered or spring water
Sweetener of choice, to taste
    (optional)

Directions:

In a large jar or pitcher, combine cherries, lime, plums, basil, and mahlab seeds, if using.

Fill the jar or pitcher with water and add sweetener if desired. Refrigerate for 3–4 hours or overnight. You may refill with water 2–3 times. Use within 2 days.

TIP

⋆Substitute mahlab seeds with raw apricot seeds or fennel seeds.

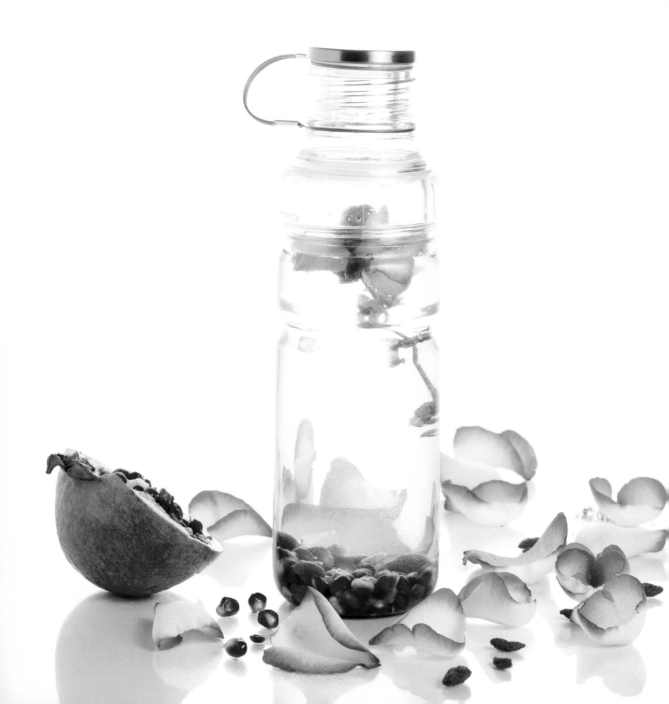

Pomegranate, Goji Berries, and Rose Water

SERVINGS: 4–6
PREP TIME: 5 MINUTES
INFUSING TIME: 3–4 HOURS

Ingredients:

⅓ cup pomegranate seeds
¼ cup dried goji berries
1 sprig fresh oregano
1–2 tablespoons rose water*
4–6 cups filtered or spring water

Directions:

In a water bottle or a jar, combine the pomegranate seeds, goji berries, oregano, and rose water and fill with water. Allow to infuse for a few hours or overnight before serving.

You may refill with water 2–3 times. Use within 2 days.

TIP
*Add a handful of pesticide-free rose petals instead of the rose water.

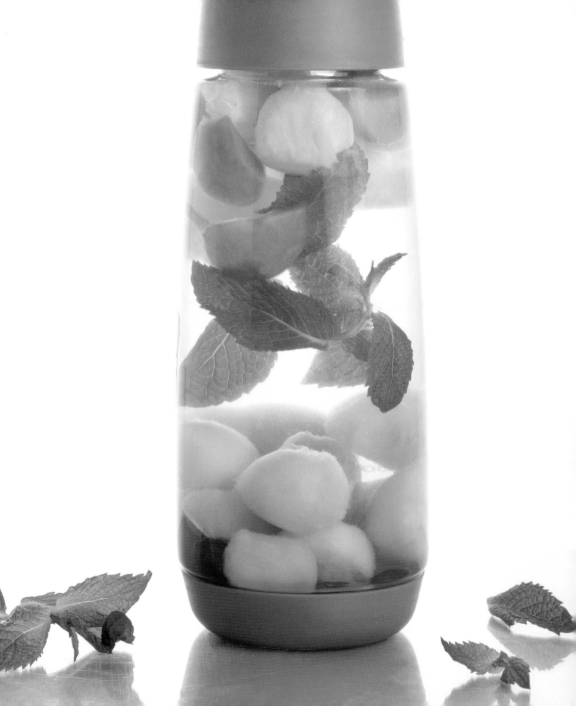

Papaya, Mango, Pineapple, and Red Grapes

SERVINGS: **4–6**
PREP TIME: **10** MINUTES
INFUSING TIME: **3–4** HOURS

Ingredients:

¼ cup each diced papaya, mango, and pineapple
⅓ cup red grapes, halved
A small handful fresh mint leaves★
1–2 lime slices, optional
4–6 cups filtered or spring water
Ice cubes, to serve

Directions:

Place all ingredients in a water bottle or a large jar and fill with water.

Allow to steep in the fridge for 3–4 hours or overnight and serve over ice.

You may refill with water a couple of times. Use within 2 days.

TIP
★Substitute mint leaves with 1–2 sprigs Thai basil.

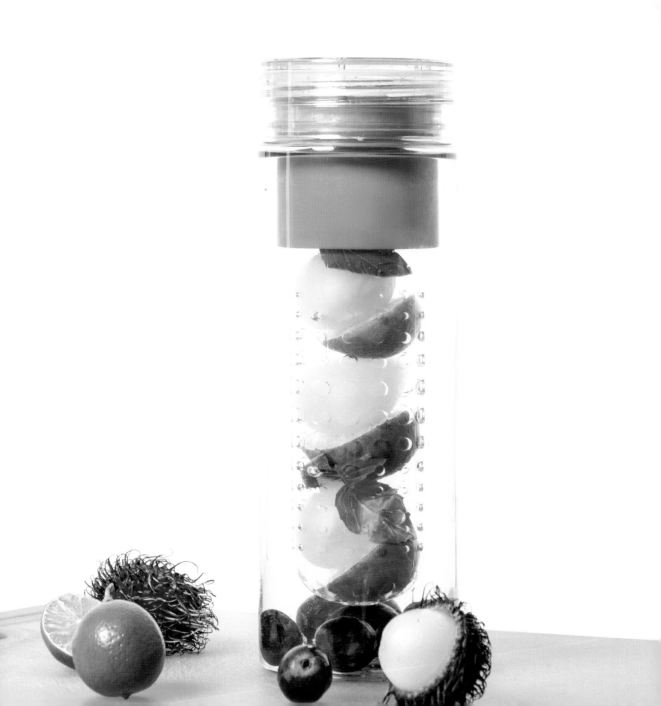

Rambutan, Key Lime, and Red Grapes

SERVINGS: 4–6
PREP TIME: 10 MINUTES
INFUSING TIME: 3–4 HOURS

Ingredients:

3–4 rambutans,* skins and seeds
  removed
3–4 key limes, halved
⅓ cup red grapes, halved
1 sprig fresh basil
4–6 cups filtered or spring water

Directions:

Add rambutans, key limes, grapes, and basil to the infuser water bottle or a jar. Pour in water and leave at least 4 hours or overnight in the refrigerator.

You can add more water and re-infuse. Drink within 2 days.

TIP
*Substitute rambutans with lychee or longan. If these tropical fruits are not available, double the quantity of the grapes.

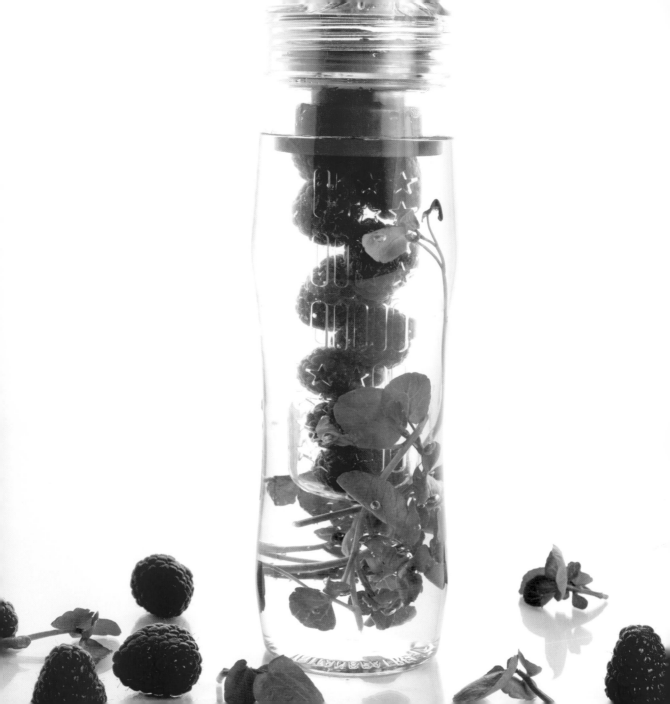

Raspberries, Watercress, and Lime

SERVINGS: 4–6
PREP TIME: 10 MINUTES
INFUSING TIME: 3–4 HOURS

Ingredients:

½ cup raspberries
1 small handful watercress
1–2 lime slices
Sweetener of choice, to taste,
    optional
4–6 cups filtered or spring water

Directions:

In an infuser water bottle, combine all ingredients and fill with water.

Chill for a few hours to allow the flavors to infuse the water and serve with ice. Use within 2 days.

TIP
Add a tablespoon of raw cacao nibs for a chocolatey taste and increased health benefits of the infused water.

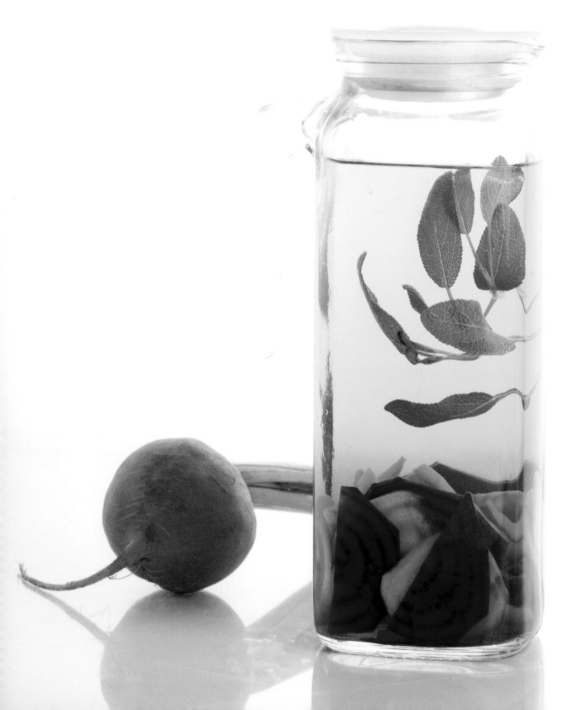

Red and Golden Beets, Pineapple, and Sage

SERVINGS: **6–8**
PREP TIME: **10** MINUTES
INFUSING TIME: **3–4** HOURS

Ingredients:

1 small red beet, trimmed, peeled, and sliced or spiralized
1 small golden beet, trimmed, peeled, and sliced or spiralized
⅔ cup pineapple slices
2 sprigs fresh sage
2–3 lime or lemon slices
6–8 cups filtered or spring water

Directions:

In a pitcher or a large jar, combine beets, pineapple, sage, and lemon. Fill with water and let infuse for 3–4 hours or overnight before serving.

Refill with water and use within 2 days.

TIP
Add a few slices of jalapeno if you enjoy a spicier taste.

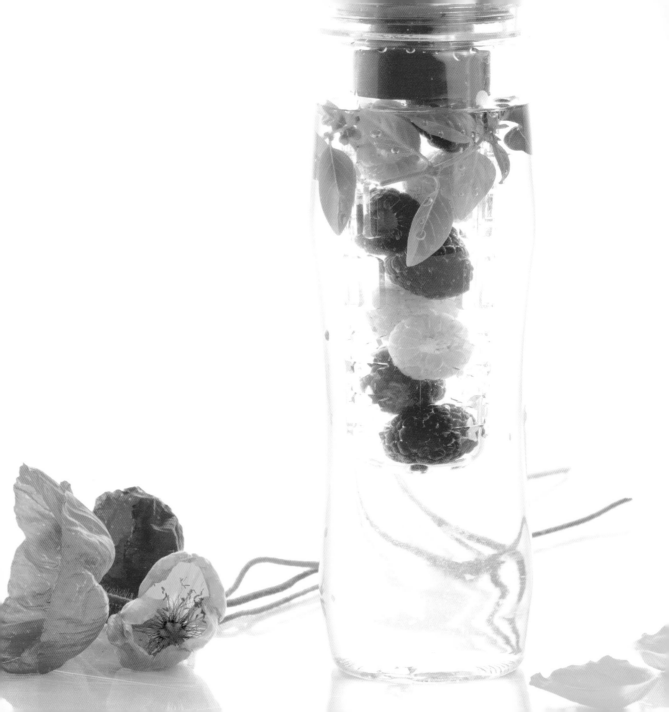

Red and Golden Berries with Basil

SERVINGS: 4–6
PREP TIME: 5 MINUTES
INFUSING TIME: 3–4 HOURS

Ingredients:

⅓ cup each golden and red
   raspberries
1–2 sprigs fresh basil*
1 lime slice
Sweetener of choice, to taste,
   optional
4–6 cups filtered or spring water

Directions:

Add raspberries, basil, and lime to an infuser water bottle and pour in water. Stir in a sweetener, if using. Leave at least 3–4 hours (or overnight for best flavor) in the refrigerator and use within 2 days.

TIP
*Omit basil and use ¼ cup of freshly made wheatgrass juice or a few edible flowers with leaves, such as poppies or pansies.

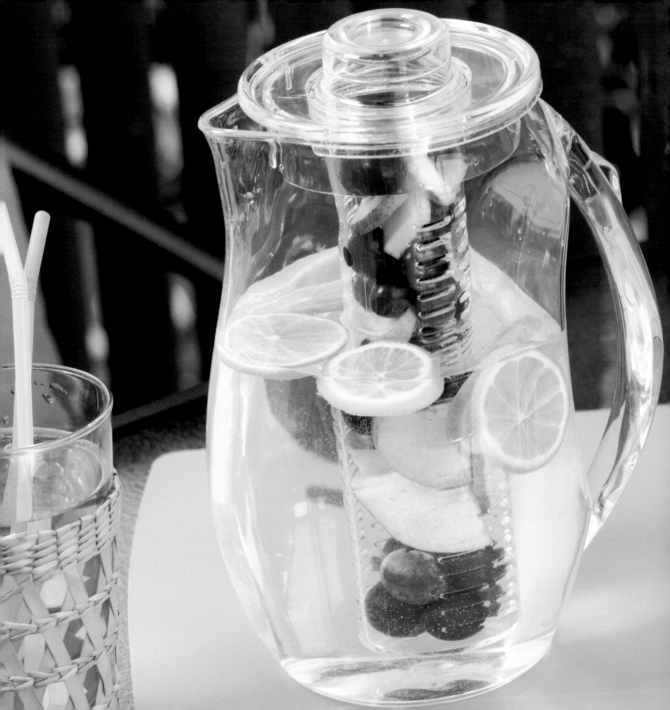

Red Grapes, Pear, and Lemon

SERVINGS: 4–6
PREP TIME: 10 MINUTES
INFUSING TIME: 3–4 HOURS

Ingredients:

¾ cup seedless red grapes, halved
1 pear, cored and sliced
1 lemon, thinly sliced
2–3 whole cloves*
6–8 cups filtered or spring water
Ice cubes, to serve

Directions:

Add grapes, pear, lemon slices, and cloves to a pitcher and fill with water.

Refrigerate overnight and serve with ice. You may refill with water 2–3 times. Use within 2 days.

TIP
*Another spice that works well with this combination is nutmeg.

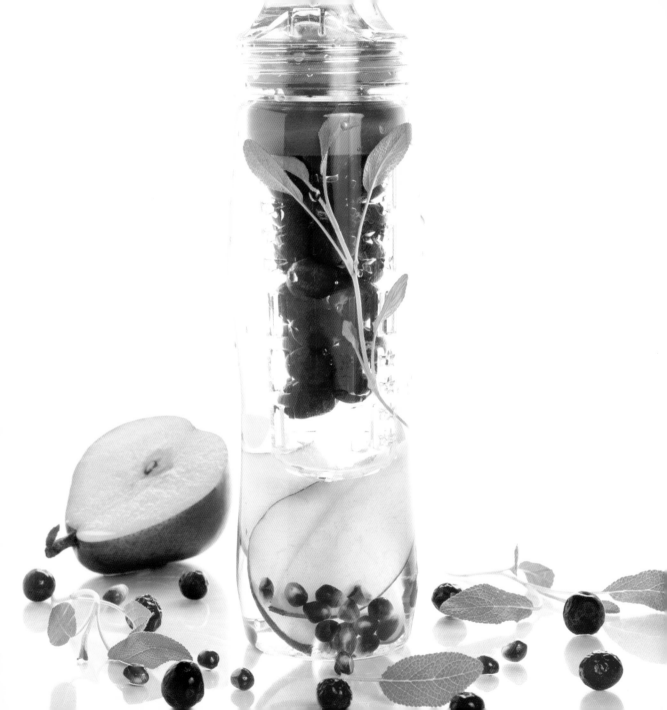

Red Pear, Cranberries, Pomegranate, and Sage

SERVINGS: 3–4
PREP TIME: 5 MINUTES
INFUSING TIME: 3–4 HOURS

Ingredients:

1 red pear, cored and sliced
1 handful fresh or frozen
   cranberries
⅓ cup pomegranate seeds
2–3 slices lime or lemon
1–2 sprigs fresh sage★
3–4 cups filtered or spring water

Directions:

Place all ingredients in an infuser water bottle and fill with water. Chill for a few hours or overnight before serving.

Refill with water once or twice and use within 2 days.

TIP
★Substitute sage with ¼–½ teaspoon fennel or anise seeds.

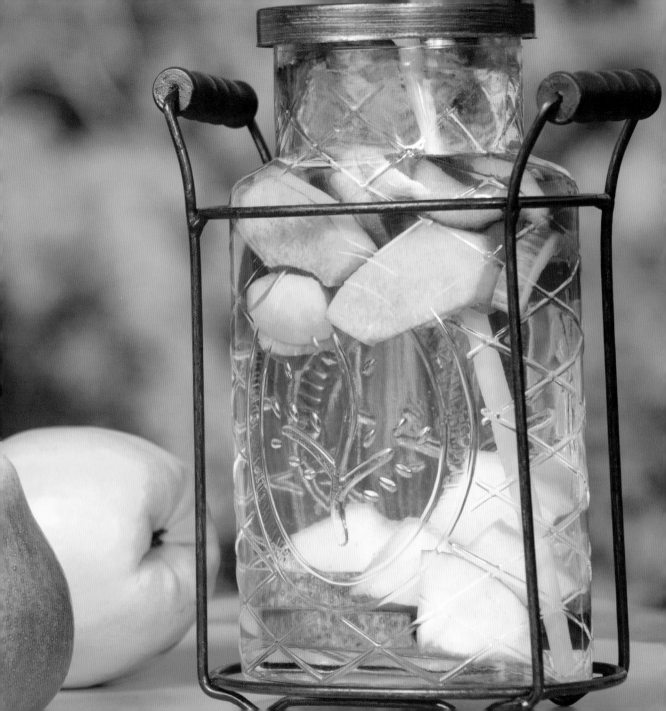

Rhubarb, Cinnamon, Quince, and Pear

SERVINGS: 6–8
PREP TIME: 10 MINUTES
INFUSING TIME: OVERNIGHT

Ingredients:

1 stalk rhubarb, sliced
1 cinnamon stick
1 quince, trimmed, cored, and sliced
1 pear, cored and sliced
1–2 tablespoons lemon or lime juice
Sweetener of choice, to taste (optional)
6–8 cups filtered or spring water

Directions:

Place the rhubarb, cinnamon, quince, pear, and lemon or lime juice in a pitcher and fill with water; stir in sweetener, if using.

Refrigerate overnight and serve. Use within 2 days.

TIP
Add a few whole allspice berries and 1 small knob of peeled and sliced fresh ginger.

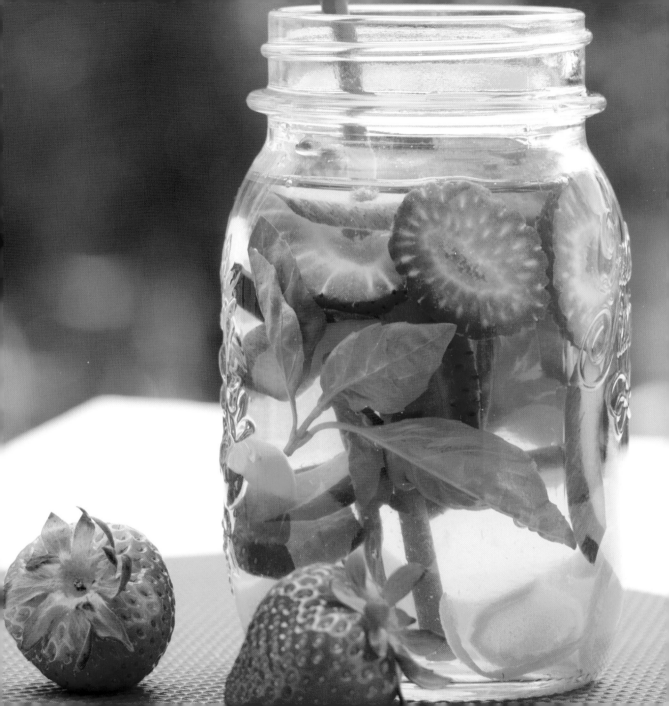

Rhubarb, Strawberry, and Ginger

SERVINGS: 4–6
PREP TIME: 10 MINUTES
INFUSING TIME: 3–4 HOURS

Ingredients:

1 rhubarb stalk, sliced
1 cup strawberries, hulled and sliced
1 (1-inch) piece fresh ginger, peeled and sliced
1–2 sprigs fresh basil
Sweetener of choice, to taste
4–6 cups filtered or spring water

Directions:

In a jar, combine all ingredients and fill with water. Let steep for a few hours or overnight. Serve chilled and use within 2 days.

TIP
Add a few tablespoons oats, 1 cinnamon stick, 1 whole nutmeg, and a vanilla bean; strain before using and serve chilled.

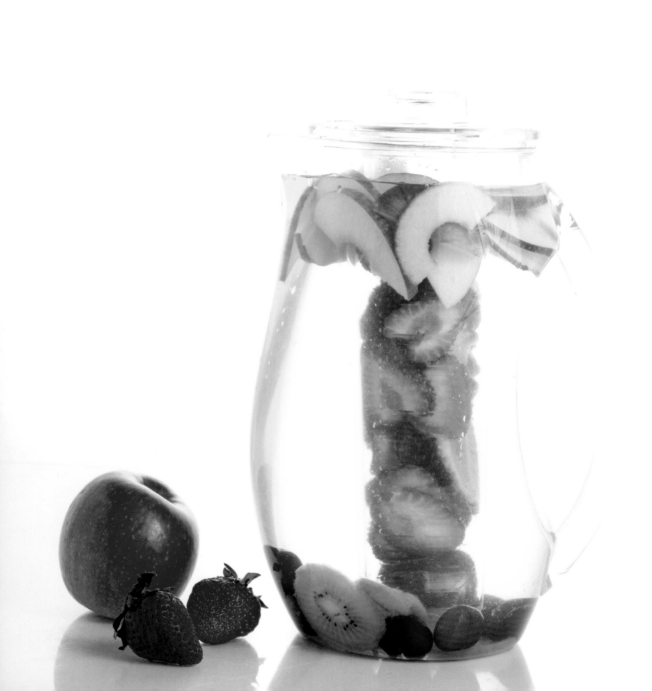

Strawberries, Apple, Kiwi, and Cherries

SERVINGS: 6–8
PREP TIME: 10 MINUTES
INFUSING TIME: 3–4 HOURS

Ingredients:

½ cup strawberries, hulled and
   sliced
1 apple, cored and sliced
1 kiwi, peeled and sliced
½ cup cherries,* pitted and halved
6–8 cups filtered or spring water
Ice cubes, to serve

Directions:

Add the strawberries, apple, kiwi, and cherries to a pitcher and fill with water. Chill for 3–4 hours or overnight and serve with ice.

Refill with water 1–2 times and use within 2 days.

TIP
*Use plums instead of cherries and add a cinnamon stick.

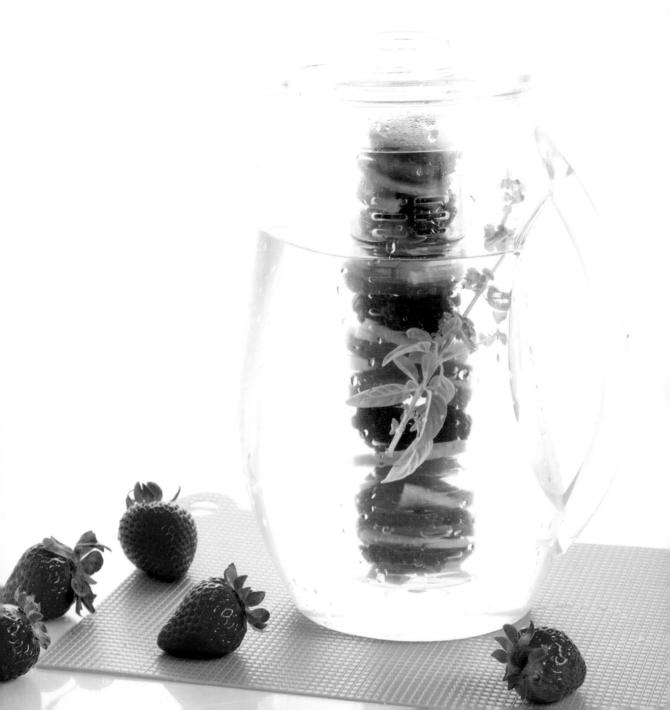

Strawberry, Blackberry, Kiwi, and Oregano

SERVINGS: 6–8
PREP TIME: 10 MINUTES
INFUSING TIME: 3–4 HOURS

Ingredients:

⅔ cup strawberries, hulled and
  sliced
⅔ cup blackberries
1 kiwi, peeled and sliced
2 sprigs fresh oregano
Sweetener of choice, to taste,
  optional
6–8 cups filtered or spring water
Ice cubes, to serve

Directions:

Combine fruit and oregano sprigs in a pitcher and fill with spring water; refrigerate for 3–4 hours to allow the flavors to infuse the water. Use within 2 days.

TIP
Create flavor variations by substituting the fresh oregano with mint or a small handful of baby arugula, and use other types of berries.

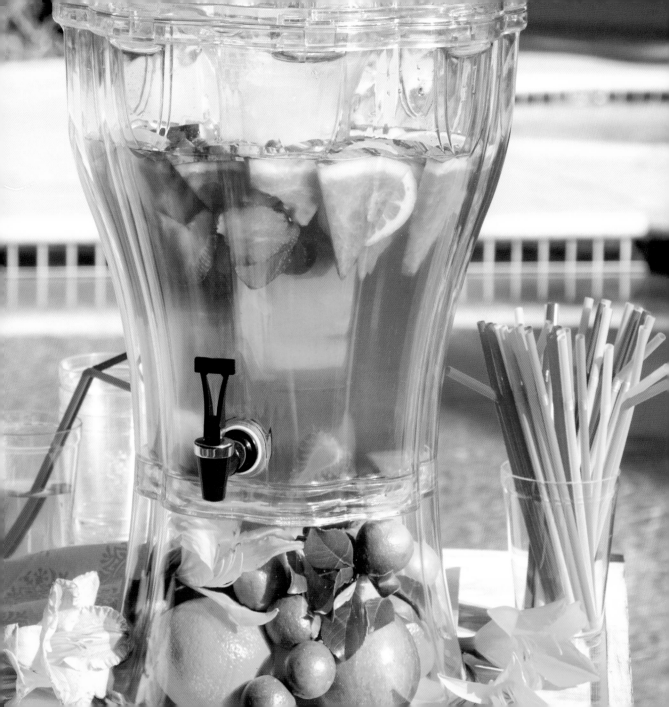

Strawberry, Cantaloupe, Watermelon, and Lemon

SERVINGS: 25–30
PREP TIME: 15 MINUTES
INFUSING TIME: 3–4 HOURS

Ingredients:

1 pound strawberries, hulled and
    halved
1–2 pounds cantaloupe, sliced or
    cubed
1–2 pounds seedless watermelon,
    sliced or cubed
2–3 handfuls fresh mint leaves*
2 Meyer lemons, thinly sliced
Ice cubes, as needed
3 gallons filtered or spring water

Directions:

Place the strawberries, cantaloupe, watermelon, mint, and Meyer lemons in a 3½ gallon beverage dispenser; add ice and fill with water.

Allow the ingredients to infuse for 2–3 hours, adding more ice as needed. Serve with ice.

Strain any leftover water into a pitcher and keep refrigerated for up to 2 days.

TIP
*Rub the fresh mint leaves lightly with your hands for a more intense flavor.

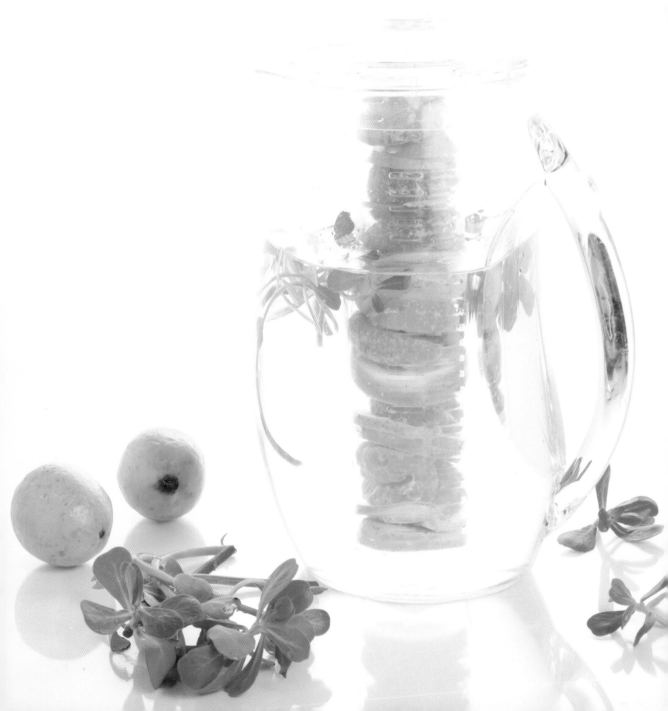

Tangerine, Guava, and Purslane

SERVINGS: 6–8
PREP TIME: 10 MINUTES
INFUSING TIME: 3–4 HOURS

Ingredients:

2 tangerines, segmented
3 guavas, trimmed and sliced
1 handful fresh purslane leaves★
1 lime, sliced (optional)
6–8 cups filtered or spring water
Ice cubes, to serve

Directions:

Combine tangerine segments, guavas, purslane, and lime, if using, in a pitcher and fill with water.

Allow to infuse for 3–4 hours in the fridge and serve with ice.

TIP
★Substitute purslane with watercress or baby kale leaves.

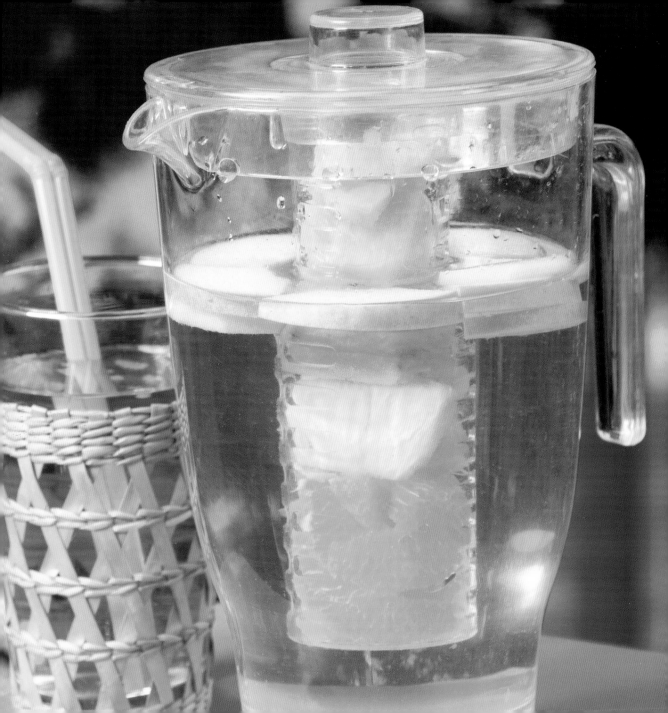

Tangerine, Pineapple, and Granny Smith Apple

SERVINGS: 6–8
PREP TIME: 10 MINUTES
INFUSING TIME: 3–4 HOURS

Ingredients:

1 tangerine, segmented
1 cup sliced or diced pineapple
1 Granny Smith apple, cored
   and sliced
2–3 lemon or lime slices
A few whole coriander seeds,
   optional
6–8 cups filtered or spring water
Ice cubes, to serve

Directions:

Combine the tangerine segments, pineapple, and apple slices in a pitcher; add lime slices and coriander seeds, if using. Fill the pitcher with water and refrigerate for at least 4 hours to allow the flavors to infuse the water. Use within 2 days.

TIP
Adding 1–2 teaspoons of orange flower water will pleasantly enhance the citrusy flavor.

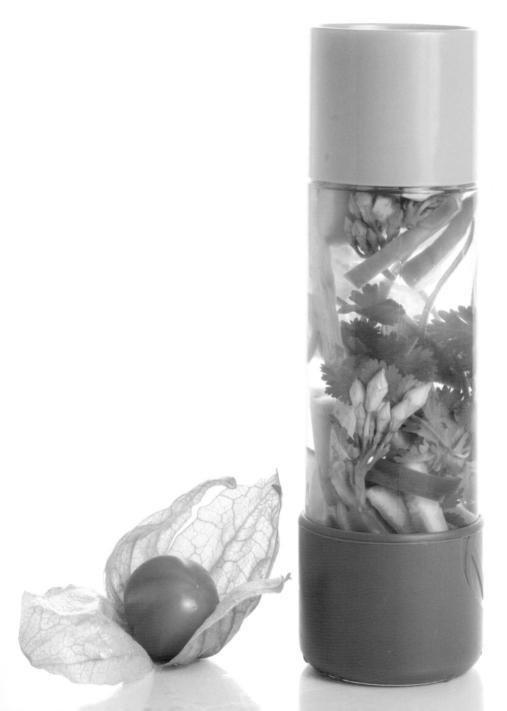

Tomatillo, Cactus Leaf, Jalapeño, and Cilantro

SERVINGS: 4–6
PREP TIME: 10 MINUTES
INFUSING TIME: 3–4 HOURS

Ingredients:

1–2 tomatillos* (husks removed), sliced
½ cup sliced cactus leaf
1 small jalapeño, seeded
A handful fresh cilantro
A few lime slices
A few loroco flower buds, optional
4–6 cups filtered or spring water
Ice cubes, to serve

Directions:

Add the ingredients to a water bottle or a jar and fill with water; refrigerate for 3–4 hours or overnight.

Keeps refrigerated for up to 2 days.

TIP

If tomatillos are not available, you may substitute with small under-ripe green tomatoes. Adding a lemon peel will further enhance the flavors.

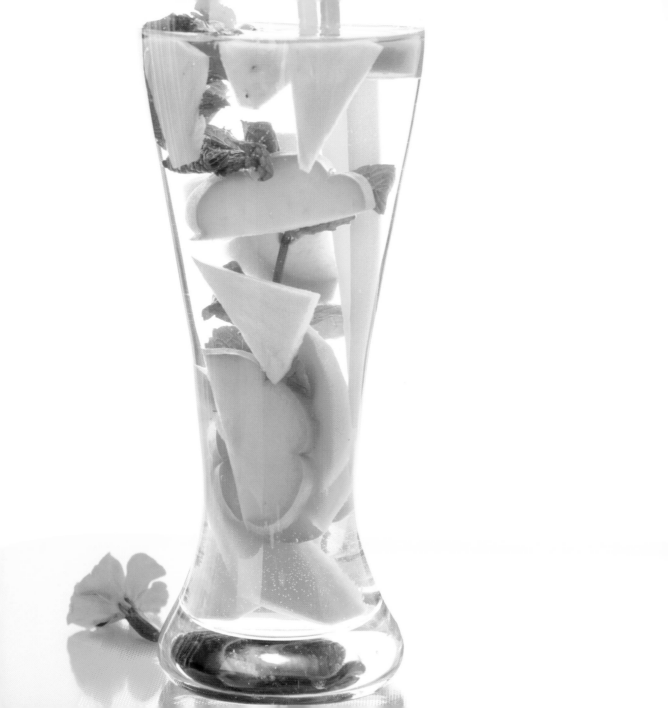

Tropical Fruit, Chayote, and Mint

SERVINGS: 6–8
PREP TIME: 10 MINUTES
INFUSION TIME: 2–3 HOURS

Ingredients:

¼ pineapple, sliced
¼ papaya, sliced
1 mango, diced
½ chayote squash,★ sliced
1 sprig mint
1–2 edible flowers (optional)
6–8 cups filtered or spring water

Directions:

Place all ingredients in a pitcher or a large glass jar.

Add water and refrigerate for about 2–3 hours before serving.

Refill with water a couple of times and use within 2 days. Keep refrigerated.

TIP
★Chayote may be substituted with sliced cucumber.

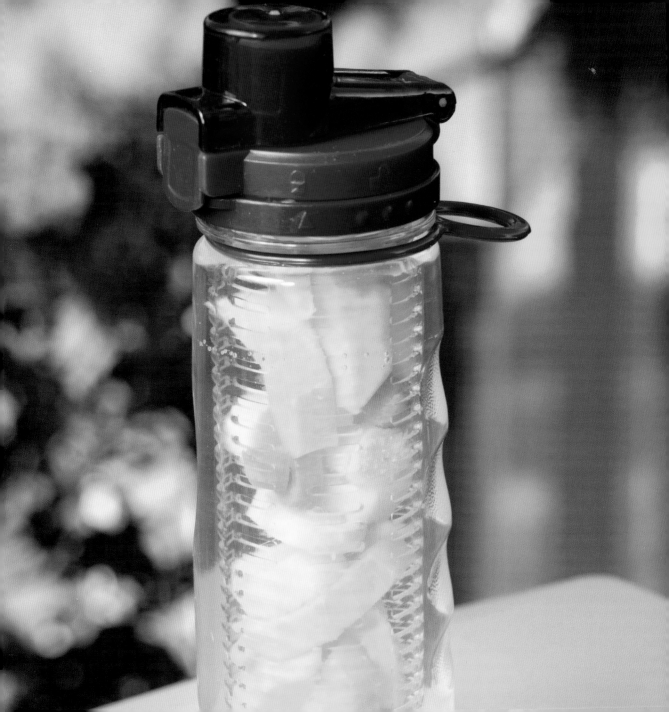

Turmeric, Ginger, Lemongrass, and Mango

SERVINGS: 4–6
PREP TIME: 10 MINUTES
INFUSING TIME: 3–4 HOURS

Ingredients:

1 (1-inch) piece fresh turmeric, peeled and sliced

1 (1-inch) piece fresh ginger, peeled and sliced

1 stalk lemongrass, tender white part only, cut into 1-inch pieces

1 mango, peeled, pitted, and sliced or diced

1 pinch cayenne pepper, optional

4–6 cups filtered or spring water

Directions:

Place sliced turmeric, ginger, lemongrass, and mango in an infuser water bottle. Add water and stir in a pinch of cayenne. Refrigerate 2–4 hours or overnight and serve with ice. Drink within 2 days.

TIP
Substitute coconut water for filtered water, or add some sliced young coconut.

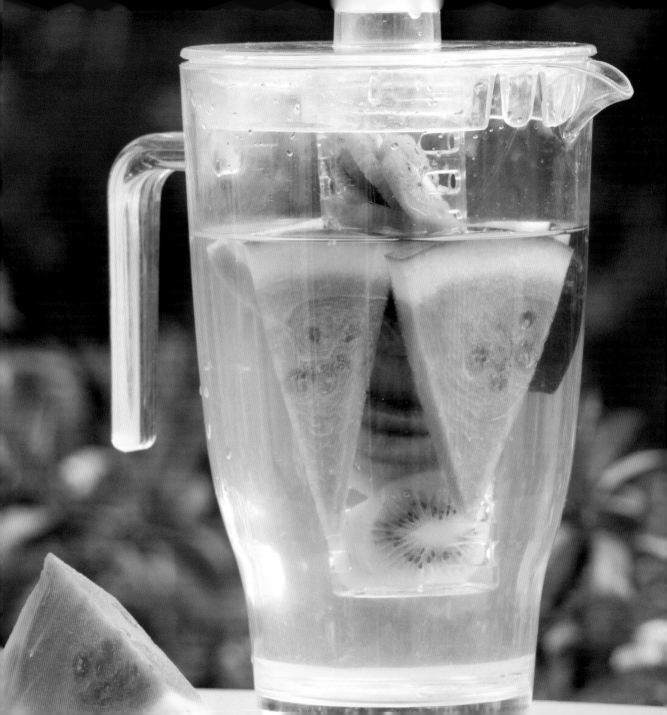

Watermelon, Kiwi, and Key Lime

SERVINGS: 4–6
PREP TIME: 10 MINUTES
INFUSING TIME: 3–4 HOURS

Ingredients:

2 cups sliced or diced watermelon
2 kiwis,* peeled and sliced
2–3 key limes, sliced
2 sprigs fresh basil, optional
6–8 cups filtered or spring water

Directions:

In a pitcher, combine watermelon, kiwis, key limes, and basil, if using. Fill the pitcher with water and refrigerate for 2–3 hours.

Serve with ice. It is best used within a day.

TIP
*Substitute kiwi with a handful of your favorite fresh or frozen mixed berries.

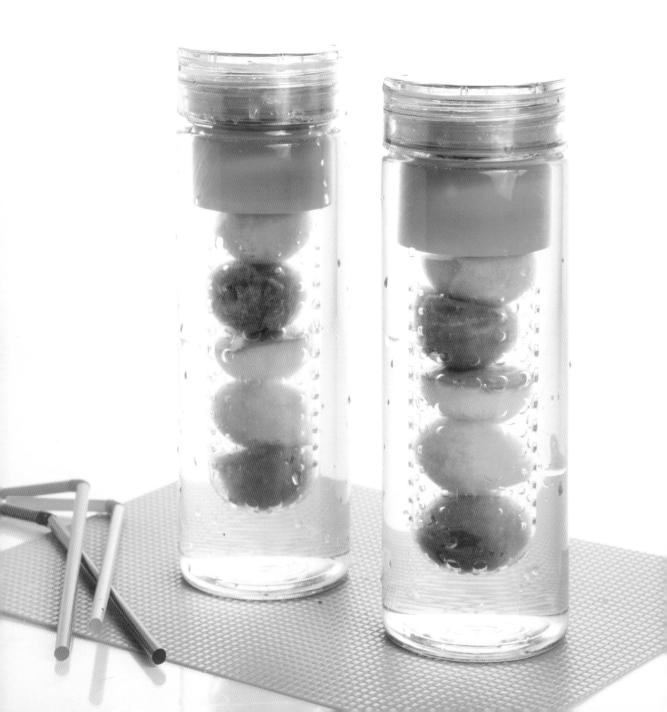

Watermelon, Chayote, and Cantaloupe

SERVINGS: 6–8
PREP TIME: 10 MINUTES
INFUSING TIME: 3–4 HOURS

Ingredients:

⅔ cup diced seedless watermelon
1 chayote, trimmed and diced
⅔ cup diced cantaloupe
2–3 tablespoons lime juice
6–8 cups filtered or spring water
Ice cubes, to serve

Directions:

Place watermelon, chayote, cantaloupe, and lime juice in a pitcher and fill with water.

Refrigerate for 2–4 hours to allow the flavors to infuse the water. Keeps in the fridge for 1–2 days.

TIP
Add a few sprigs of fresh mint or basil.

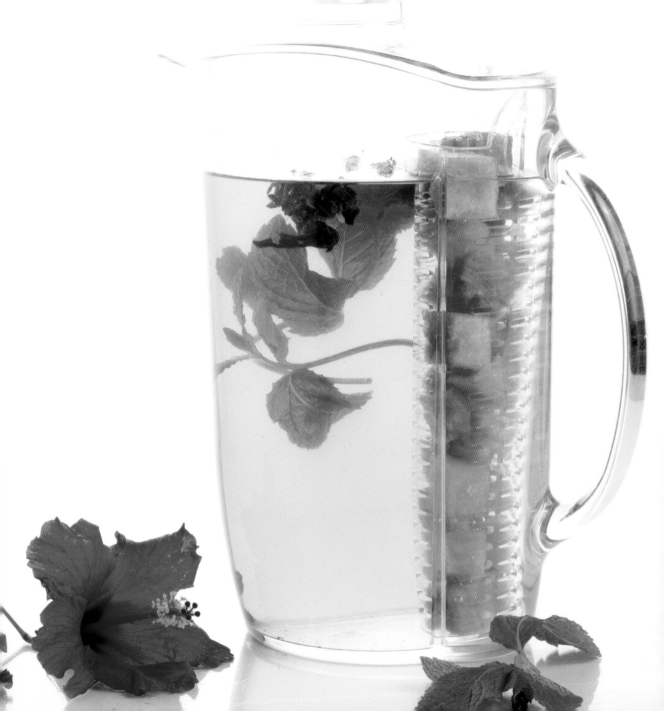

Watermelon, Hibiscus, and Mint

SERVINGS: 6–8
PREP TIME: 10 MINUTES
INFUSING TIME: 3–4 HOURS

Ingredients:

1½ cup diced seedless watermelon
1–2 tablespoons dried hibiscus
   flowers
2–3 sprigs fresh mint
1 slice of lemon
6–8 cups filtered or spring water
Ice cubes, to serve

Directions:

Place watermelon, hibiscus, mint, and lemon in a pitcher. Fill the pitcher with spring water and refrigerate for about 4 hours to allow the flavors to infuse the water.

You may refill with water 2–3 times. Use within 2 days.

TIP
Substitute dried hibiscus flowers with 2–3 bags hibiscus tea and add 1 tablespoon dried goji berries.

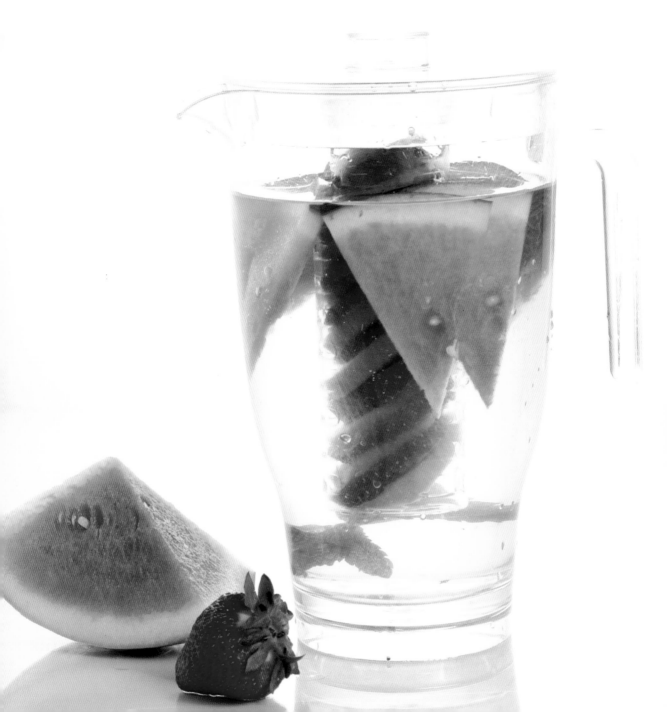

Watermelon, Strawberry, Kiwi, and Mint

SERVINGS: 6–8
PREP TIME: 10 MINUTES
INFUSING TIME: 2–4 HOURS

Ingredients:

- ½ cup strawberries, hulled and sliced
- 2 kiwis, peeled and sliced
- ½ lime, sliced
- 6–7 seedless watermelon slices, about ½-inch thick
- 2–3 sprigs fresh mint★
- 6–8 cups filtered or spring water

Directions:

Place strawberry, kiwi, and lime slices in the flavor infuser. Add watermelon and mint and fill the pitcher with water.

Refrigerate for 2–4 hours (or overnight) to allow the flavors to infuse the water. Serve over ice, if desired. Use within 24 hours.

TIP
★Substitute fresh mint with other fresh herbs, such as parsley or basil.

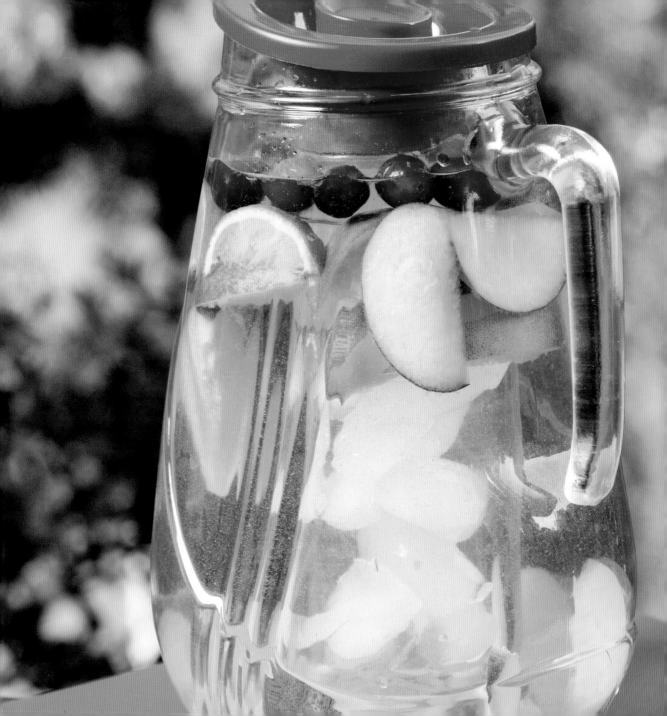

White Peach, Apricot, Nectarine, and Cranberries

SERVINGS: 4–6
PREP TIME: 10 MINUTES
INFUSING TIME: 3–4 HOURS

Ingredients:

1 white peach, stoned and sliced
2 apricots, stoned and sliced
1 nectarine, stoned and sliced
½ cup fresh or frozen cranberries
1–2 lime or lemon slices
1 (1½-inch) piece cinnamon bark
  (optional)
6–8 cups filtered or spring water
Ice cubes, to serve

Directions:

Combine peach, apricots, nectarine, cranberries, and lime or lemon slices in a pitcher; fill with water and allow to steep for at least 4 hours or overnight.

Keep refrigerated and use within 2 days.

TIP
Make this infused water with only one type of stone fruit, for example, plums, and substitute cinnamon with a vanilla bean.

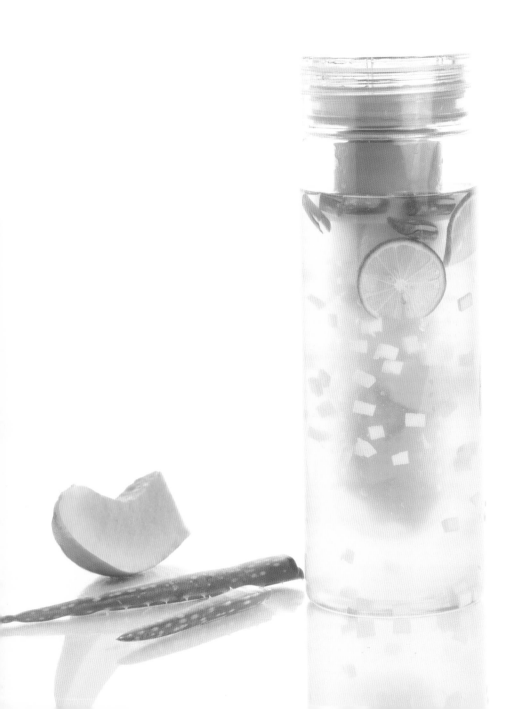

Young Coconut, Mango, Papaya, and Aloe Vera

SERVINGS: 4–6
PREP TIME: 10 MINUTES
INFUSING TIME: 3–4 HOURS

Ingredients:

1 young coconut
½ cup diced mango
½ cup diced papaya
1 tablespoon food-grade aloe vera gel
2–3 lime slices
3–4 cups filtered or spring water, as needed

Directions:

Carefully cut the young coconut open and reserve the water, then scoop out the flesh and dice.

In an infuser water bottle, combine diced coconut, mango, papaya, aloe vera gel, and lime slices. Add the reserved coconut water, top with filtered water, and stir.

Refrigerate for 3–4 hours or overnight and use within 2 days.

TIP
Add a cored and sliced Asian pear and a few leaves of purple basil.

Index